The 7-Day Gluten Free Diet Plan

35 Healthy Wheat Free Recipes To Banish Your Wheat Belly

Volume 1

By Rachel Richards

© Revelry Publishing 2015

Copyright 2015 by Revelry Publishing

All Rights reserved under International and Pan-American Copyright Conventions. By payment of required fees, you have been granted the non-exclusive, non-transferable right to access and read the text of this book. No part of this text may be reproduced, transmitted, downloaded, decompiled, reverse-engineered or stored in or introduced into any information storage and retrieval system, in any form or by any means, whether electronic or mechanical, now known, hereinafter invented, without express written permission of the publisher.

DISCLAIMER

Every effort has been made to ensure that the information in this book is accurate and complete. However, the author and the publisher do not warrant the accuracy of the information, text and graphics contained within the book due to the rapidly changing nature of science, research, known and unknown facts and the internet. The author and the publisher do not hold any responsibility for errors, omissions or contrary interpretation of the subject matter herein. This book is presented solely for motivational and informational purposes only.

Nutritional values have been calculated with due care and attention. However, there may be differences in the calorie count due to the variance of each individual kitchen creation caused by ingredient amounts, brand differences, different cuts and quality of meats etc. The nutritional values of these recipes are provided as a guideline only.

ISBN-13: 978-1987863154
ISBN-10: 1987863151

Other books by Rachel Richards:

The 7-Day Ketogenic Diet Meal Plan: 35 Delicious Low Carb Recipes For Weight Loss Motivation - Volume 1

The first volume of the set contains 35 different recipes and a bonus of a recipe for 'Keto Rolls'.

The 7-Day Ketogenic Diet Meal Plan: 35 Delicious Low Carb Recipes For Weight Loss Motivation - Volume 2

The second volume of the set contains 35 different recipes and a bonus of a recipe for 'Keto Almond Bread'.

The 7-Day Ketogenic Diet Meal Plan: 35 Delicious Low Carb Recipes For Weight Loss Motivation - Volume 3

The third volume of the set contains 35 different recipes and a bonus of a recipe for 'Posh Coffee'.

The 7-Day Ketogenic Diet Meal Plan: 35 Delicious Low Carb Recipes For Weight Loss Motivation - Volumes 1 to 3

This book has all three volumes of the set containing 105 different recipes and their respective bonuses of recipes for 'Keto Rolls', 'Keto Almond Bread' and 'Posh Coffee'.

50 Vegan Slow Cooker Recipes: Delicious Meatless Slow Cooker Meals For The Vegan Lifestyle

This book was written for those who enjoy a Vegan lifestyle or just want a meatless meal from time to time.

Get the latest update on new releases from the author at:

https://rachelrichardsrecipebooks.com/newsletter

Volume 1

Table of Contents

Introduction 1
Shopping List 4
Bonus 9
The 7-Day Meal Plan Table 10
DAY 1 11
    Gluten-Free Crepes 12
    Tomato and Mint Dip 14
    Radicchio Cups with Prawns and Mango 16
    Thai Steak Salad 18
    Chocolate Almond Pudding 20
DAY 2 22
    Herby Corn Fritters with Avocado Salsa 23
    Oven Baked Fries 25
    Orange Spiced Chicken 27
    Pork Steaks with Fennel, Orange and Apple 29
    Maple and Star Anise Roasted Plums 31
DAY 3 33
    Spinach and Tomato Breakfast Cup 34
    Mexican Chicken Nachos 36
    Chicken, Prawn and Chorizo Paella Style 38
    Basque-style Salmon Stew 40
    Gluten-Free Brownies 42
DAY 4 44
    Honey Apple Yogurt 45
    Cranberry and Raspberry Smoothie 47
    Middle Eastern Salad with Grilled Halloumi 49
    Salmon Scallion and Ginger Fishcakes 51
    Lemon Tart with Fresh Blueberries 53
DAY 5 56
    Easy Scrambled Eggs 57
    Sausage Rolls with a Kick! 59
    Pancetta and Polenta Bake 61
    Oriental Lamb Stir Fry 63
    Mango and Papaya Fool 65

DAY 6 67
- Stuffed Herb Mushrooms.. 68
- Fig and Pistachio Flapjacks 70
- Lemon and Herb Salmon 72
- One Pot Beef Stew 74
- Mixed Berry Bake.. 76

DAY 7 78
- Cheesy Scones 79
- Provence Pizza 81
- Homemade Savory Crackers... 84
- Chinese Pork Tenderloin with Braised Cabbage and Leek 86
- No Bake Coconut Cookies 88

Thank You! 90
Other Books by Rachel Richards... 91
About the Author – Rachel Richards 92
Connect with Rachel Richards... 93

Introduction

Why gluten-free?

Perhaps you are suffering from a wheat-intolerance, celiac disease or simply wanting to cleanse your system or even embark on a weight loss diet. There are many reasons, including childhood problems such as autism and ADHD, but these are more complex than just practicing a gluten-free lifestyle.

The desire for following a diet of this kind is growing on a daily basis, for all the above reasons. Many people are under the misconception that a gluten-free diet will be restrictive, not tasty and hard to follow. You couldn't be more wrong!

Other than baking, the list of foods available to you is vast – you will be able to pick and choose from a huge variety of foods that will keep your interest at optimum level and you will never feel that you are missing anything. Not only that, all those nasty symptoms you experience with gluten intolerance will disappear quite rapidly.

Symptoms

Symptoms vary from person to person and can be quite violent or at the other end of the spectrum, just something that is a nuisance on a daily basis.

Most commonly, the symptoms are gastrointestinal, but those suffering with a severe gluten intolerance problem will find that many other parts of their body or system react violently to the presence of gluten in any foodstuffs.

Bloating, diarrhea or constipation and headaches are the most common, followed by fatigue, skeletal pain and anaemia. As a person suffering from gluten intolerance, you may also experience dermatitis herpetiformis (DH), which manifests itself by itchy and even blistered skin.

Continued intolerance without diagnosis can result in damage to the intestines, so it is best if you suffer from any of the symptoms that you get checked out by your health practitioner as soon as possible.

Are there any pitfalls in following a gluten-free diet?

Nutritionists advise that overall a gluten-free diet should not harm you, and that the only deficiency you may suffer from is lack of Vitamin B and fiber, which are contained in most grains. This can be substituted by supplements, or indeed, other grains that are gluten-free but have high levels of Vitamin B and also protein. In this instance, the best grains are amaranth, oats, quinoa and teff. Other vitamins and minerals are found in abundance in fruit, vegetables and of course meat and fish, particularly oily fish.

What to do to get started

The first port of call is to empty your cupboards, fridge and freezer of any products that may contain gluten. Remove any sweet temptations in particular. There is no use in thinking 'oh, just one biscuit won't hurt me' – it almost certainly will if you are truly gluten intolerant. Even if you have products that you have looked at and are sure are gluten-free, you should still remove them. Culprits are items that include sauces and mayonnaise – you may well have made a sandwich with these, using bread that is not gluten-free, but the jar you dipped into may well have been contaminated. So rid yourself of any open jars, pots or tubs that you may have used.

You must sanitize to remove any possible traces of gluten on your work surfaces, fridge, preparation equipment, pots and pans. There could be a major issue of cross-contamination, so all equipment and surfaces should be thoroughly scrubbed with hot soapy water, and if available, a sanitizer. Remember every item, from rolling pins to toasters, chopping boards to cake tins and muffin pans. Everything! This is not so easy if you are cooking or preparing for others, but it can be done by sectioning off cupboards that contain only the equipment you need to use – the rest can go in a communal storage space.

Shopping

Get into the habit of checking every label. When items are marked 'gluten-free' (there is usually a gluten-free section in most supermarkets) you should be relatively safe, but it does not hurt to still check. Quite a few products that are purportedly gluten-free, may contain a trace that could affect you. Processed foods and some sauces may contain gluten, even though they could be on a list of non-gluten products – check the labels. If you don't understand what is on the label, put it back on the shelf and pick another!

Plan your outing to the supermarket, and if at all possible, try to shop separately for your gluten-free produce. It is easy to get confused when you are shopping for multi-purpose products, and one or two may slip into your cupboards!

The Recipes

The recipes have been kept slightly below the RDA (recommended daily allowance) in terms of calorie intake, to allow you to have a 'little more' food on certain courses, or an extra small snack. For women, the RDA for calories is 1500 kcal, and for men 2000 kcal. If you are trying to lose weight as well as cut out gluten for health purposes, this will enable you to have a slow but steady weight loss without feeling too hungry, nothing dramatic. But do feel free to move the recipes around to accommodate your tastes, whilst still keeping on or below the RDA.

A few of the recipes will have more than 4 servings – but most of these can be frozen for use another day, or consumed as another snack the next day.

Shopping List

Store Cupboard

- Salt
- Ground black pepper
- All purpose flour (gluten-free)
- Bicarbonate of soda
- GF baking powder
- Vegetable oil
- Olive oil
- Sesame oil
- Honey
- Flaked almonds
- Maple syrup
- Caster sugar
- GF icing sugar
- Brown sugar
- Butter
- Flaked almonds
- Star anise
- Cinnamon powder
- Cinnamon sticks
- Cumin seeds
- Vanilla extract
- Ground almonds
- Cocoa powder
- Agave syrup
- Apple cider vinegar
- Smoked paprika
- Dried thyme
- Quick cook basmati rice
- GF vegetable stock
- GF beef stock
- GF chicken stock
- Peanut butter
- Tamari/soy sauce (GF)
- Dijon mustard
- Sherry
- Red wine
- Dried oregano
- Dried thyme
- Dried rosemary
- Bay leaves
- Chinese five-spice powder
- Chai seeds
- Ground saffron/turmeric
- Red pepper flakes
- Weekly List
- Dairy
- 30 eggs
- 1 pint milk
- 2 packs butter

The 7-Day Gluten-Free Diet Plan

Vegetables and Fruit

- 4 white onions
- 8 red onions
- 3 bulbs garlic
- 1 head celery
- 2 carrots
- 6 limes
- 6 lemons

Day 1

- 3 radicchio heads
- 9oz/250g cooked and peeled king prawns
- 3 medium to large mangos
- 1 carton salad cress
- 2 x 7oz/200g sirloin steaks (thin cut or 'bash' them out to thin as possible)
- 1 bag mixed green leaves
- Bunch Thai basil
- Small sprig fresh coriander
- Large handful mange tout peas

Day 2

- 1 can sweet corn
- Bunch parsley
- Bunch chives
- 6 red potatoes
- 1½oz/45g Parmesan cheese
- 1lb/450g boneless chicken breasts
- 1lb/450g tomatoes
- 2 large handfuls of fresh baby spinach leaves
- 1 orange
- 2 large fennel bulbs or 4 baby fennel bulbs
- 1 red apple
- 1 small orange
- Small bunch rosemary
- 4 x 7oz/200g pork steaks (lean as possible)
- 1 bag baby spinach
- 1½lb/675g plums, or a mix of plums, greengages and mirabelles
- 2 large oranges
- Mascarpone or Greek yogurt, to serve

Day 3

- 1 bag spinach (9oz/250g)
- 3 x 14oz/400g can chopped tomatoes
- Small bunch fresh basil
- 1 bag tortilla chips
- 2 cooked chicken breasts, shredded
- 1 bunch scallions
- 2 small red chillies
- 6oz/170g reasonably strong colored cheddar
- 2 avocados
- 5 bell peppers, any color
- 7oz/200g raw prawns, peeled and deveined
- 8oz/225g basmati rice (quick cook)
- 3oz/85g cooked chorizo
- Small bunch parsley
- 14oz/400g baby potatoes
- 4 salmon fillets (4-5oz/115-150g)
- 14oz/400g can black beans

Day 4

- 8fl.oz/250ml Greek Yogurt (whole milk)
- 2 crisp apples
- 2½oz/75g dates
- 6½fl.oz/200ml cranberry juice
- 1 bag frozen raspberries
- 6.5fl.oz/200ml natural yogurt
- Small bunch fresh mint
- 1 red pepper
- 1 green pepper
- 1 pack quinoa
- Small bunch flat-leaf parsley
- 10oz/300g halloumi cheese
- 2 x 5oz/140g skinless salmon fillets
- 1 large sweet potato
- 1 bunch scallions
- 4fl.oz/120ml thick cream

Day 5

- 1 large tomato
- Herbs to garnish (should be some left from previous days)

The 7-Day Gluten-Free Diet Plan

- 1 block gluten-free puff pastry
- 8 gluten-free sausages
- Small bunch parsley
- Small bunch sage
- 1 red chilli
- 5oz/140g pancetta or lardons (cubed)
- Small bunch fresh thyme
- 2oz/55g fresh Parmesan cheese
- 5fl.oz/150ml single cream
- 9oz/250g ready cooked polenta

- 1lb/450g lamb steak, sliced
- 1 red pepper
- 1 bunch spring onions (scallions)
- 8oz/225g baby sweetcorn
- 8oz/225g mange tout peas
- 8oz/225g bean sprouts
- 1 large mango
- 1 large papaya
- 5fl.oz/150mls low fat Greek Yogurt

Day 6

- 4oz/115g (dairy free) butter
- 8 large flat mushrooms
- 3½oz/100g fresh white gluten-free breadcrumbs
- Small bunch thyme
- Small bunch parsley
- 5oz/140g dried figs (you could also use dried apricots or other dried fruit)
- 6oz/170g gluten-free rolled oats

- 3oz/85g pistachio nuts
- 4 x salmon fillets (approximately 4oz/115g each)
- 2 large potatoes, cut into 1inch/2cm chunks
- 8fl.oz/240ml red wine
- 1¾lb/800g mixed berries (frozen)
- 1oz/25g flaked almonds or other nuts that you enjoy
- Small bunch fresh dill
- 1lb/450g stewing beef

Day 7

- Carton of buttermilk (or use milk from weekly shop)
- 4oz/115g cheddar or 2oz/55g cheddar and

2oz/55g Parmesan (extra cheesy taste if you combine)

- 1 x ¼oz/7g sachet fast action yeast

- 1tsp xanthan gum
- 2 large sweet white onions, or 3 medium size red onions
- 4 bell peppers, mixed
- Small jar baby gherkins
- Jar olives
- 6oz/170g strong cheddar cheese, grated (or half cheddar, half Parmesan)
- 4 shallots
- ¼ cup dry white wine
- 1 large leek
- 1 green cabbage
- 12oz/340g crushed pineapple
- 1lb/450g cream cheese
- 1lb/450g coconut flakes

Bonus

As a perk for purchasing this book, you can get two additional recipes (Braised Lamb Shanks with Butternut Squash and Gluten-Free Flour Mix), a printable meal plan and shopping list by visiting the link below:

https://gotorecipecookbooks.com/gluten-free-1/

If you enjoyed the recipes in this book, please take a moment to leave a review at your favorite retailer.

Thank you for trying out this meal plan book.

Good luck!

The 7-Day Meal Plan Table

7-day meal plan

	DAY 1	DAY 2	DAY 3	DAY 4	DAY 5	DAY 6	DAY 7
Breakfast	Gluten free crepes	Herby corn fritters and avocado salsa	Spinach and tomato breakfast cup	Honey and apple yogurt	Easy scrambled eggs	Stuffed herb mushrooms	Cheesy scones
Snack	Tomato and mint dip	Oven baked fries	Mexican chicken nachos	Cranberry and raspberry smoothie	Sausage roll with a kick	Fig and pistachio flapjack	Provencal pizza
Lunch	Radicchio cups	Orange spiced chicken	Chicken, prawn and chorizo paella style	Middle Eastern salad and halloumi	Pancetta and polenta bake	Lemon and herb salmon	Homemade crackers x 4
Dinner	Thai steak salad	Pork steaks with fennel and apple	Basque style salmon stew	Salmon, scallion and ginger fishcake	Oriental stir fry	One pot beef stew	Chinese pork tenderloin with cabbage and leeks
Dessert	Chocolate almond pudding	Maple and star anise roasted plums	Gluten free brownie	Lemon tart with blueberries	Mango and papaya fool	Mixed berry bake	No bake coconut cookies
Daily Calories:	1451	1263	1652	1463	1467	1737	1597

DAY 1

Gluten-Free Crepes

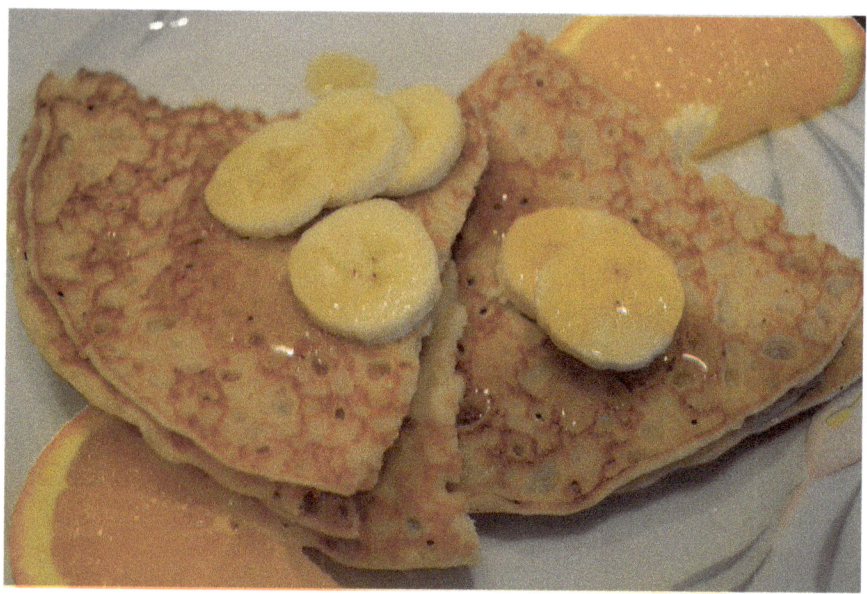

These crepe-style pancakes are light but filling. Use a little honey, chopped banana or fresh fruit to serve a delicious breakfast.

Servings: 8 small pancakes
Preparation Time: 5 minutes
Cooking Time: 25 minutes plus resting

Ingredients:

- 5oz/140g gluten-free plain flour
- 1 egg
- 8fl.oz/250ml milk
- butter, for frying

Method:

1. Put the flour in a bowl and make a well in the center.
2. Crack the egg in the middle and pour in about a quarter of the milk. Use an electric or balloon whisk to thoroughly combine the mixture.
3. Once you have a paste like consistency and it will be very thick, mix in another quarter and once lump free, mix in the remaining milk. Leave to rest for 20 minutes. Stir again before using.
4. Heat a small non-stick frying pan with a knob of butter.
5. When the butter starts to foam, pour a small amount of the mixture into the pan and swirl around to coat the base – you want a thin layer.
6. Cook for a few minutes until golden brown on the bottom, then turn over and cook until golden on the other side.
7. Repeat until you have used all the mixture, stirring the mixture between pancakes and adding more butter for frying as necessary.
8. Use greaseproof paper to keep the pancakes separated.
9. Serve with raw honey and a squeeze of orange juice or your pancake filling of choice.

Fresh berries are always a perfect pairing for crepes.

Nutritional Values	per Serving (2)
Calories	346
Protein	8g
Fat	22g
Carbs	31g

Tomato and Mint Dip

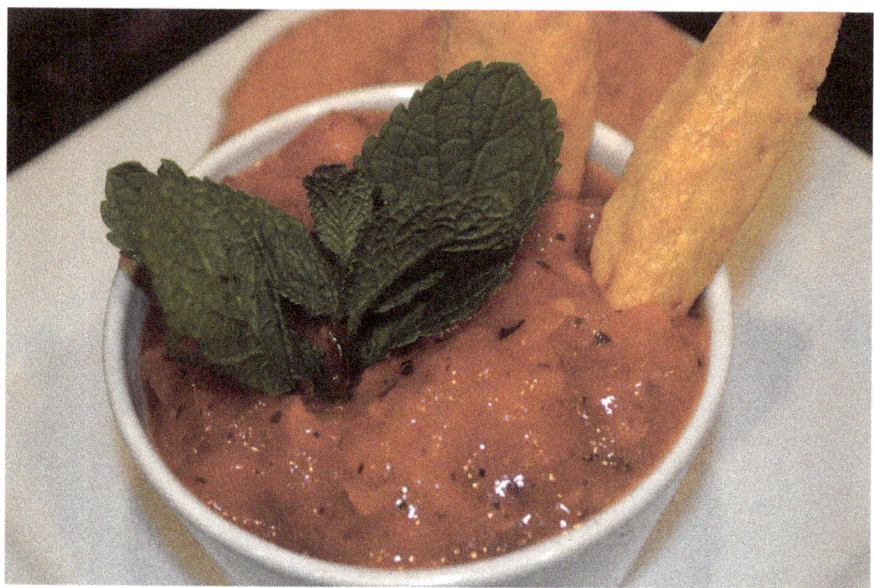

This is a great dip to serve with gluten-free crackers. The danger is you will eat too many of the crackers with this as it is deliciously spicy and 'moreish'. When making this, if you want a 'chunkier' salsa style dip, only blitz for a little time, so that you leave some of the onions intact.

Servings: Approximately 1 cup of dip
Preparation Time: Less than 5 minutes
Cooking Time: No cooking required

Ingredients:

- 2½oz/75g tomatoes, cut into quarters
- 2½oz/75g red onion, chopped
- 2½oz/75g fresh mint leaves
- 2½oz/75g fresh coriander leaves
- 2 green chilies, finely chopped
- 2tbsp lime juice

- salt to taste

Method:

1. Blend all the ingredients in a blender till well blended or lightly pulse or blitz for a shorter time to achieve a more chunky dip.
2. Serve with crudités or gluten-free crackers (remember to add the calorie intake for the crackers).

Nutritional Values	per Whole Cup
Calories	109
Protein	6g
Fat	1g
Carbs	23g

Radicchio Cups with Prawns and Mango

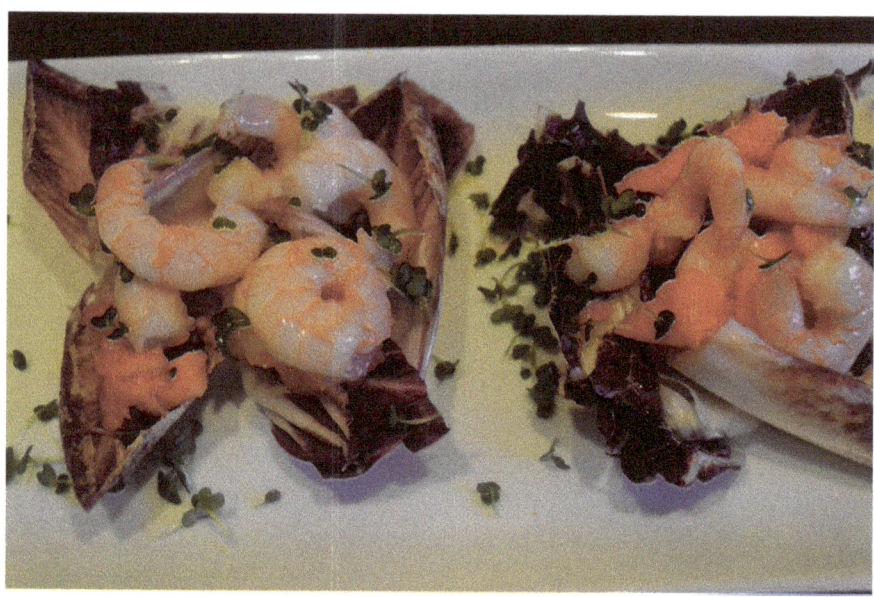

Juicy prawns pair beautifully with sweet mango and crunchy, slightly bitter leaves in this simple lunch dish, finished with lemon juice and coriander.

Servings: 8 portions (2 each)
Preparation Time: 20 minutes
Cooking Time: No cooking required

Ingredients:

- 3 radicchio heads
- 9oz/250g cooked and peeled king prawns
- 3 medium to large mangos, peeled, de-stoned and diced
- 1 carton salad cress
- 3tbsp olive oil
- Juice 2 lemons and rind of 1 lemon, grated
- 2tsp finely chopped coriander

Method:

1. Separate the radicchio heads into leaves choosing the best ones, then divide the king prawns, mango pieces and a few sprigs of salad cress between them.
2. Assemble a few hours ahead and chill.
3. Whisk together the olive oil, lemon juice and finely chopped coriander and drizzle a little over each filled radicchio leaf.

Nutritional Values	per Serving (2 each)
Calories	314
Protein	11g
Fat	12g
Carbs	42g

Thai Steak Salad

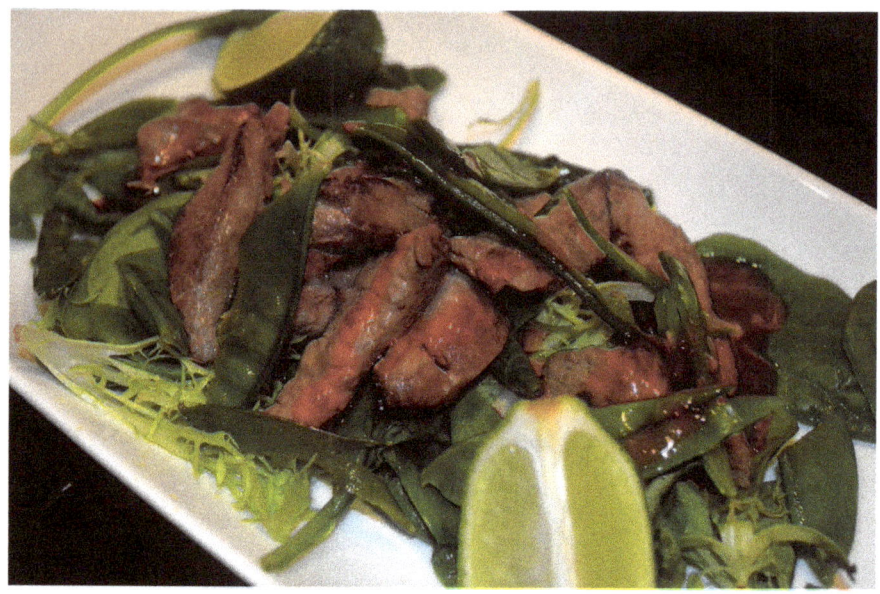

A really quick lunch or supper dish if you prefer, with delicious Thai herbs and spices to bring out the flavor.

Servings: 4
Preparation Time: Less than 5 minutes
Cooking Time: 2-3 minutes

Ingredients:

- 2 x 7oz/200g sirloin steaks (thin cut or 'bash' them out to thin as possible)
- 2tbsp olive oil
- 5oz/140g mixed green leaves (you can normally find these in your supermarket)
- Large handful Thai basil, roughly chopped
- Juice and zest of 2 limes
- 1tbsp fresh garlic, minced

- 2tsp tamari sauce (most tamari sauce is gluten-free, but check the label)
- Large handful mange tout peas, sliced into strips
- Ground black pepper to taste

Method:

1. Mix together the lime juice, zest, garlic and tamari sauce.
2. Rub the olive oil and ground black pepper into the steaks.
3. Heat a griddle pan or frying pan until almost smoking, then cook the steaks on each side for 2 minutes, so that they are still slightly pink in the middle. Remove to rest.
4. Mix together all the salad ingredients.
5. Slice the steak diagonally into strips and place on the top of the salad.
6. Pour over the dressing and serve, the steak should still be slightly warm.

Nutritional Values	per Serving
Calories	210
Protein	17g
Fat	13g
Carbs	7g

Chocolate Almond Pudding

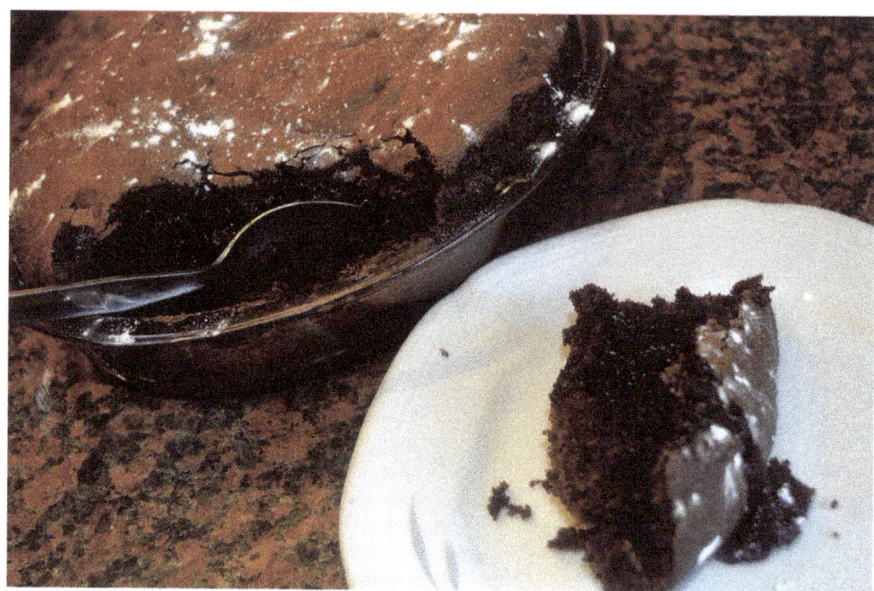

These are so delicious and look like you have taken hours to make them. You could also serve them with a chocolate or caramel sauce, to make them even more decadent! The recipe is for 2 darioles, but double the quantity and make one whole pudding, as shown!

Servings: 2 (double quantities for 4 molds or 1 round dish)
Preparation Time: 10 minutes
Cooking Time: 20-25 minutes

Ingredients:

- 2oz/55g butter, softened, plus extra for the molds
- 2oz/55g caster sugar
- 1 egg
- 1oz/25g gluten-free flour
- 1oz/25g ground almonds
- 1tbsp cocoa powder
- Extra cocoa powder for dusting dariole molds

Method:

1. Heat oven to 325°F/160°C/gas mark 3.
2. Butter 2 x 5fl.oz/150ml (or one small oval baking dish) dariole molds, and dust the insides with the extra cocoa powder. Place on a small baking tray.
3. Beat the butter, sugar, egg, flour, ground almonds and cocoa powder together, then divide between the molds.
4. Bake for 20-25 minutes until a skewer comes out clean (The large dish will probably need 30 minutes – test in the centre and if a skewer comes out clean then the pudding is cooked).
5. Leave to cool until safe to handle and then run a knife around the inside of the dariole molds.
6. Turn upside down on separate plates and tap the mold. The chocolate pudding should come out cleanly.
7. Serve with delicious creamy vanilla ice cream!

Nutritional Values	per Serving
Calories	472
Protein	8g
Fat	32g
Carbs	42g

DAY 2

Herby Corn Fritters with Avocado Salsa

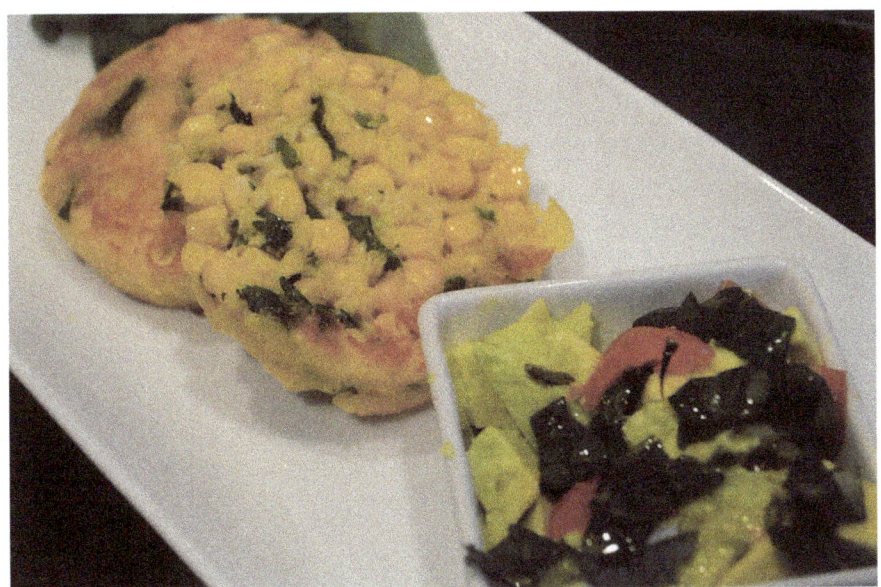

These are pretty tasty for breakfast, or you could have them for brunch or lunch. You could also substitute the corn for some crispy, crunchy bacon.

Servings: 8 fritters (2 each)
Preparation Time: 10 minutes
Cooking Time: 10 minutes

Ingredients:

- 4oz/115g gluten-free plain flour
- 1tsp bicarbonate of soda
- 2 eggs
- 14oz/400g canned sweetcorn
- 3tbsp fresh herbs, finely chopped (chives, parsley are good for this dish)
- Oil for frying (vegetable is probably best)

For the salsa

- 2 avocados, skinned, de-stoned and cut into small chunks
- 2 medium sized tomatoes, seeds removed and cut into small chunks

- Juice of 1 lime
- Seasoning to taste

Method:

1. Mix the flour, bicarbonate of soda, eggs and a little seasoning in a bowl.
2. Heat the oil in a non-stick frying pan.
3. Drop 1tbsp (heaped) of the corn mix into the pan, leaving spaces between each one you drop. Press the droplets down firmly to make them more 'patty-like'.
4. Cook for 2 or 3 minutes on each side until golden and crispy. You may need to do this in two batches, so keep the first batch warm.
5. Whilst the fritters are cooking, make the salsa by mixing together the avocado, herbs and tomatoes.
6. Mix in the lime juice and season well.

Enjoy!

Nutritional Values	per Serving (2 each)
Calories	395
Protein	11g
Fat	20g
Carbs	47g

Oven Baked Fries

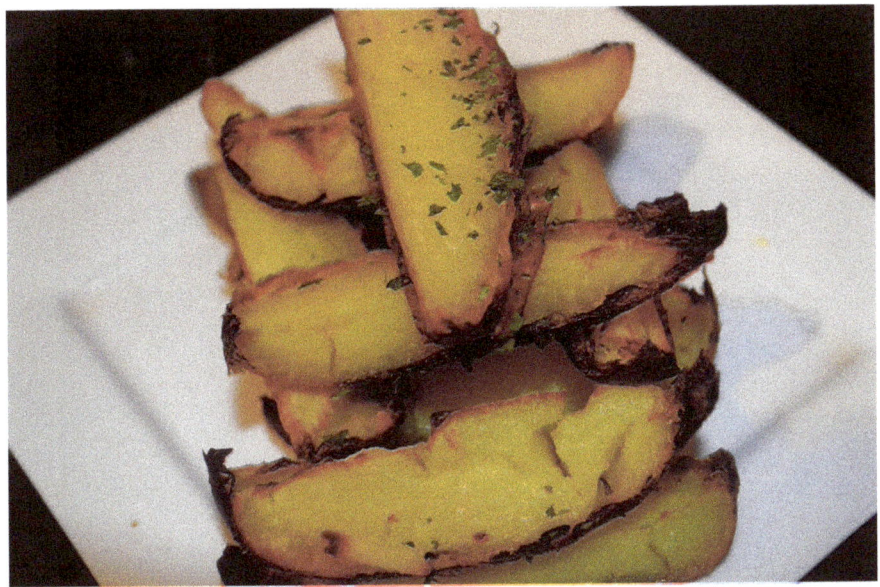

Fries are always something that everyone enjoys, so make these when you have people over to watch a football match or any other get-together!

Servings: 6 (equally divided)
Preparation Time: 10 minutes
Cooking Time: 30 minutes

Ingredients:

- 6 red potatoes, well washed
- 1½oz/45g Parmesan cheese
- 1½tbsp olive oil
- 1½tsp oregano
- 3tsp basil
- 1½tsp garlic powder
- Salt to sprinkle over when cooked

Method:

1. In a bowl, mix Parmesan cheese, olive oil, oregano, basil, and oregano.
2. Cut potatoes into long slices and mix them with the cheese mixture.
3. Transfer the potatoes onto a greased baking sheet and bake for at 425°F/220°C/Gas mark 7 for 15 minutes, then turn the potatoes and bake for a further 15 minutes.
4. Test for tenderness.
5. Bake for a few more minutes if still a little hard.

Serve and enjoy.

Nutritional Values	per Serving
Calories	212
Protein	6g
Fat	6g
Carbs	36g

Orange Spiced Chicken

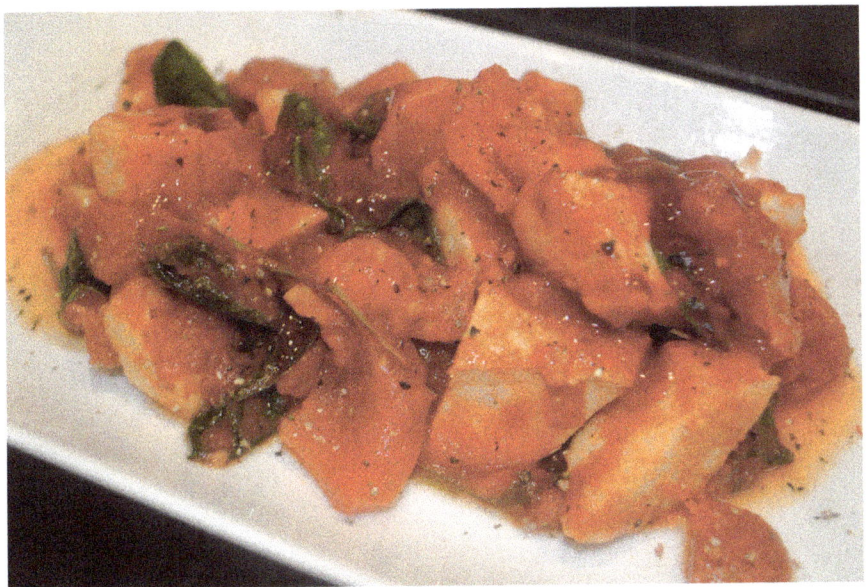

This is a very simple dish to make. If you are working all day, this can also be cooked in the slow cooker for 5-6 hours, by simply adding some more liquid and seasoning (makes no difference to calorie intake).

Servings: 4
Preparation Time: 5 minutes
Cooking Time: 30 minutes maximum

Ingredients:

- 1lb/450g boneless chicken breasts, cut into medium sized chunks
- 1tsp crushed red pepper
- 1tsp agave syrup
- 1lb/450g tomatoes (diced)
- 2 large handfuls of fresh baby spinach leaves
- ½tsp black pepper
- 2tbsp apple cider vinegar
- Salt to taste
- Zest of 1 orange, grated

Method:

1. Marinate chicken with all the ingredients (except spinach) for at least half an hour.
2. Place in a non-stick pan and cook on medium heat for 20 minutes and check to see how the chicken is cooking. If still slightly pink, continue to cook for a further 5 minutes.
3. If you need more liquid, gradually add a little water until desired consistency is reached.
4. Finally add the spinach leaves, stir in and place a lid over the top of the pan (If you don't have a lid, cover with aluminum foil).
5. Turn off the heat and leave the dish to steam so that the spinach cooks through.
6. Serve with a little brown rice or a mixed bell pepper salad.

Nutritional Values	per Serving
Calories	172
Protein	26g
Fat	4g
Carbs	8g

Pork Steaks with Fennel, Orange and Apple

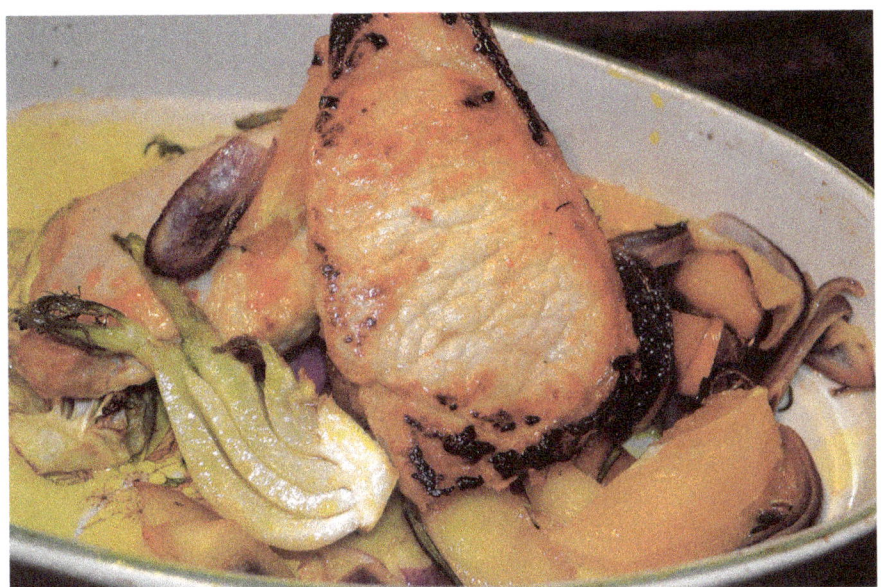

If you like the sweetness of fruit with pork, then this dish is sure to please.

Servings: 4
Preparation Time: 15 minutes
Cooking Time: 25 minutes

Ingredients:

- 2 large fennel bulbs or 4 baby fennel bulbs, trimmed, thickly sliced
- 2 small red onions, cut into wedges
- 1 red apple, cored, cut into wedges
- 1 small orange, peeled and segmented
- 1 tbsp apple cider vinegar
- 2 tbsp olive oil
- 1 tbsp rosemary leaves, roughly chopped
- 4 x 7oz/200g pork steaks (lean as possible)
- 2 large handfuls baby spinach

Method:

1. Preheat the oven to 400°F/200°C/Gas mark 6.
2. Toss the fennel, onion, orange and apple with the vinegar and 1tbsp of the olive oil in a large flameproof/ovenproof skillet.
3. Sprinkle with rosemary and season with salt and pepper.
4. On a low heat with the lid on the pan, cook for 15 minutes or until the fennel and onion are tender.
5. Turn off the heat.
6. Season the pork steaks all over with ¼tsp sea salt each and freshly ground black pepper.
7. Heat the remaining oil in a frying pan over high heat. When very hot, cook the pork steaks for 3 minutes each side or until brown.
8. During last 5 minutes of vegetable cooking time, put the pork in with the vegetables and transfer the whole dish to the oven to finish cooking.
9. Remove the dish from the oven, add the spinach and toss gently to combine (this should wilt the spinach but still leave it fairly fresh).
10. Serve vegetables topped with pork and drizzled with pan juices.
11. You may like to add braised red cabbage as a side dish.

Nutritional Values	per Serving
Calories	234
Protein	14g
Fat	11g
Carbs	23g

Maple and Star Anise Roasted Plums

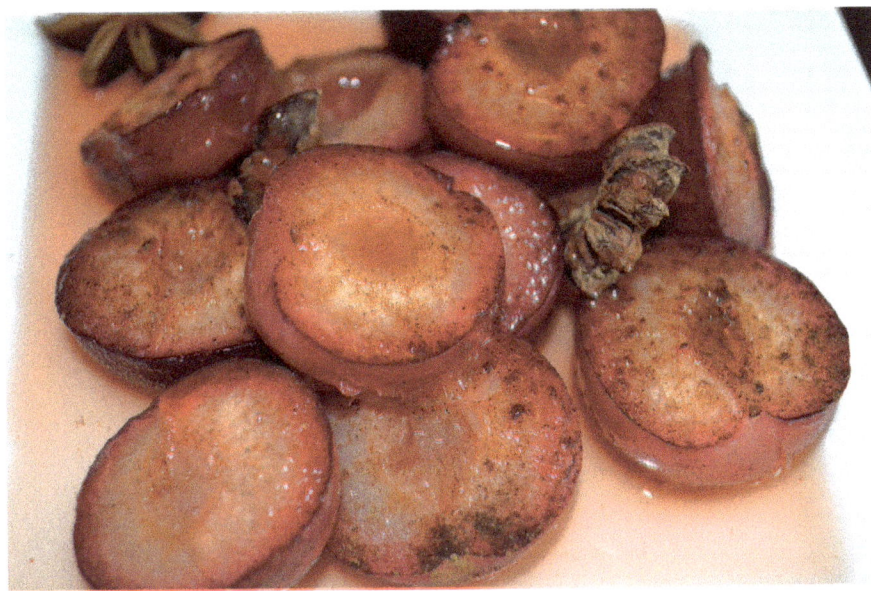

You can use just one variety of plum for this simple dessert, or choose a mixture of colors and flavors - it's up to you.

Servings: 4
Preparation Time: 25 minutes
Cooking Time: 50 minutes

Ingredients:

- 1½lb/675g plums, or a mix of plums, greengages and mirabelles
- Juice 2 large oranges
- 3 star anise
- 2 sticks cinnamon
- 3-4tbsp maple syrup
- Mascarpone or Greek yogurt, to serve

Method:

1. Heat oven to 350°F/180°C/Gas mark 4.
2. Arrange the plums in a single layer in a 35fl.oz/1-liter gratin dish.
3. Pour over orange juice, tuck star anise among the plums, drizzle over the maple syrup, then gently stir.

4. Bake for 30-35 minutes until the fruit is soft but not collapsed.
5. Serve warm or cold with mascarpone or yogurt on the side.
6. The roasted plums can be kept in the fridge for up to 3 days.

Nutritional Values	per Serving
Calories	188
Protein	8g
Fat	1g
Carbs	41g

DAY 3

Spinach and Tomato Breakfast Cup

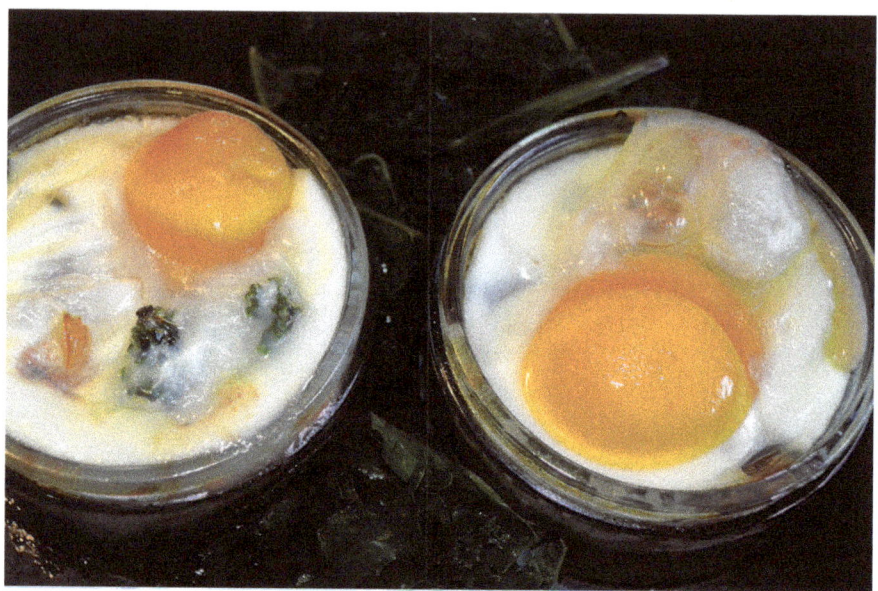

A quick and simple dish (you could actually get it ready for baking the night before). This dish is low in calories, so you could eat 2 of these quite easily!

Servings: 4
Preparation Time: 5 minutes
Cooking Time: 15 minutes

Ingredients:

- 3½oz/100g bag spinach
- 14oz/400g can chopped tomatoes
- 4 eggs
- Small handful fresh basil, chopped
- Seasoning to taste

Method:

1. Heat oven to 400°F/200°C/Gas mark 6.
2. Put the spinach into a colander then pour over a kettle of boiling water to wilt the leaves. Squeeze out excess water.
3. Mix the chopped basil through the spinach and season with salt and pepper. A little grated nutmeg is also a delightful addition.
4. Mix the tomatoes with some seasoning then add to the dishes with the spinach.
5. Make a small well in the center of each and crack in an egg.
6. Bake for 12-15 minutes or more depending on how you like your eggs.
7. Serve with gluten-free bread, if you like, or add a slice of crispy bacon.

Nutritional Values	per Serving (1 each)
Calories	97
Protein	8g
Fat	5g
Carbs	5g

Mexican Chicken Nachos

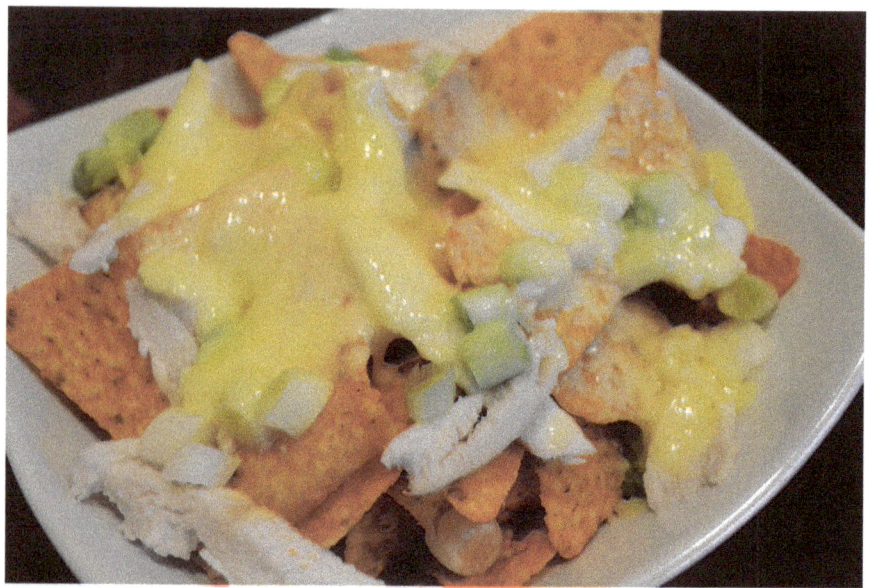

A great 'by the TV' snack, which doesn't take much time at all. Good recipe for the family to enjoy and for you to serve up quickly!

Servings: 4 (equally divided)
Preparation Time: Less than 5 minutes
Cooking Time: 8-10 minutes

Ingredients:

- 7oz/200g plain or spicy gluten-free tortilla chips
- 2 cooked chicken breasts, shredded
- 8 scallions, finely sliced
- 2 small red chillies, very finely sliced
- 6oz/170g reasonably strong colored cheddar
- 2 avocados, mashed to serve as a dip (you can add a little hot sauce if required, or some mashed garlic and seasoning)

Method:

1. Heat oven to 350°F/180°C/Gas Mark 4.
2. Layer up the tortilla chips, chicken, scallions, chilli and cheese in an ovenproof dish.
3. Bake in the oven for 8-10 minutes until cheese is bubbling.
4. For extra flavor, you could add some chopped fresh coriander and a squeeze of lime

Eat as fast as you can – they will get a little soggy after too long!

Nutritional Values	per Serving
Calories	733
Protein	43g
Fat	44g
Carbs	42g

Chicken, Prawn and Chorizo Paella Style

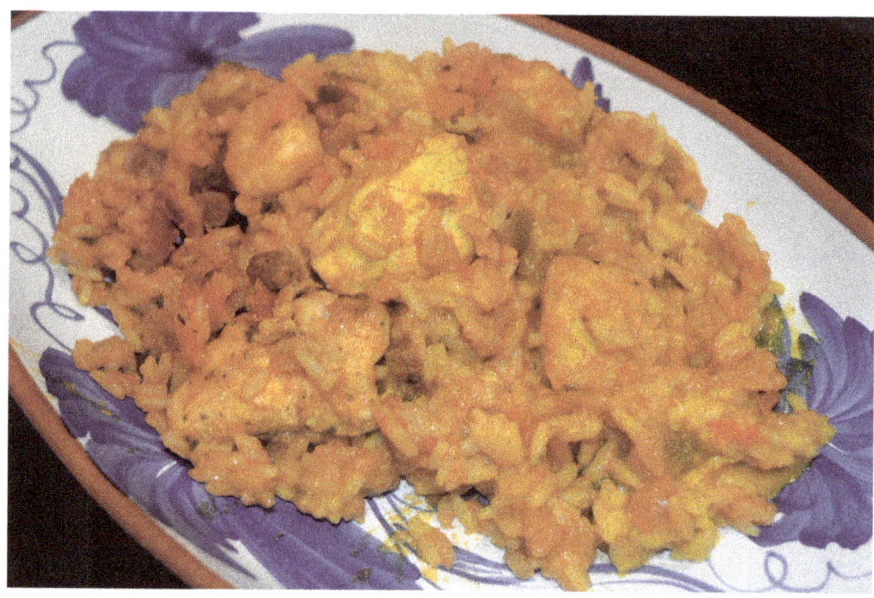

Lovely dish, smacking of Spanish flavors and a filling dinner or supper dish. Great for a party or large numbers as it is easy to make and can be done in one cooking pot!

Servings: 4
Preparation Time: 10 minutes
Cooking Time: 15-20 minutes

Ingredients:

- 2tbsp olive oil
- 1 Spanish onion (these are usually white and sweeter)
- 2 bell peppers, any color, sliced into strips
- 2 garlic cloves, crushed (if you like garlic, add more!)
- 7oz/200g raw prawns, peeled and deveined
- 14oz/400g can chopped tomatoes, preferably sugar-free
- 8oz/225g basmati rice (quick cook)
- 16fl.oz/480ml gluten-free vegetable stock

- 3oz/85g cooked chorizo, sliced into rounds
- 2 pinches ground saffron (expensive but worth it! – you could use turmeric)
- Parsley to garnish (chopped)

Method:

1. If you have a two-handled pan, this is great as you can serve the dish straight to the table.
2. Heat the oil and put the onion, chorizo, garlic and peppers into the pan. Stir continuously.
3. Add the rice and chopped tomatoes, plus the saffron or turmeric. Stir, add stock.
4. Cover the pan with a lid, but if you don't have one, use foil to seal the top of the pan.
5. Cook for 15 minutes.
6. Test the mix. The rice should be cooked and tender.
7. Stir in the raw prawns and a little water and continue to cook for 1-2 minutes until the prawns are pink and cooked through.
8. Serve straight to the table with a side salad or some gluten-free crusty bread.

A taste of Spain!

Nutritional Values	per Serving
Calories	453
Protein	18g
Fat	16g
Carbs	59g

Basque-style Salmon Stew

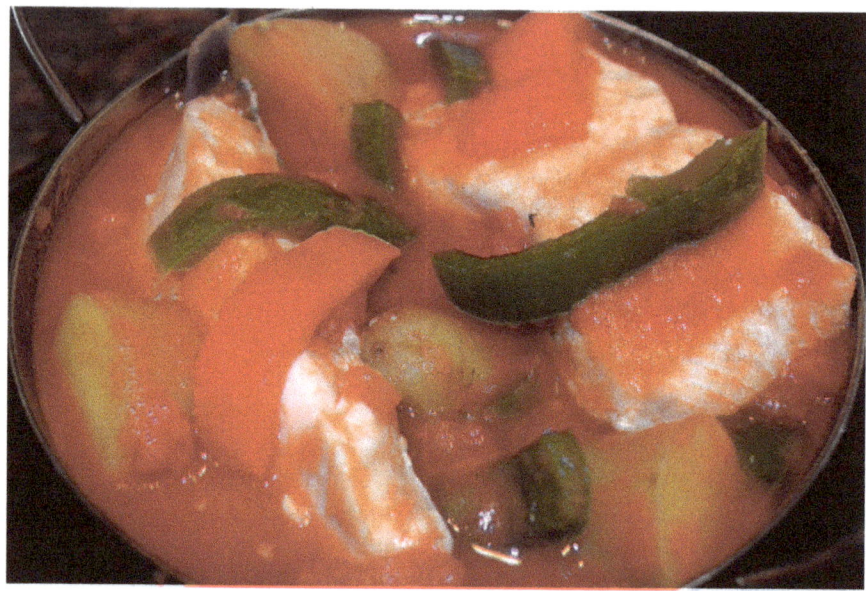

Heart-healthy salmon tops this simple one-pot dish which will help towards your five-a-day

Servings: 4
Preparation Time: 10 minutes
Cooking Time: 25 minutes

Ingredients:

- 1tbsp olive oil
- 3 mixed peppers, deseeded and sliced
- 1 large onion, thinly sliced
- 14oz/400g baby potatoes, unpeeled and halved
- 2tsp smoked paprika
- 2 garlic cloves, sliced
- 2 tsp dried thyme
- 14oz/400g can chopped tomatoes
- 4 salmon fillets (4-5oz/115-150g)

- 1tbsp chopped parsley, to serve (optional)

Method:

1. Heat the oil in a large pan and add the peppers, onion and potatoes.
2. Cook, stirring regularly for 5-8 minutes until golden.
3. Add the paprika, garlic, thyme and tomatoes.
4. Bring to a boil, stir and cover, then turn down heat and simmer for 12 minutes.
5. Add a splash of water if the sauce becomes too thick.
6. Season the stew and lay the salmon on top, skin side down.
7. Place the lid back on and simmer for another 8 minutes until the salmon is cooked through.
8. Scatter with parsley, if you like, and serve.

Nutritional Values	per Serving
Calories	335
Protein	28g
Fat	11g
Carbs	32g

Gluten-Free Brownies

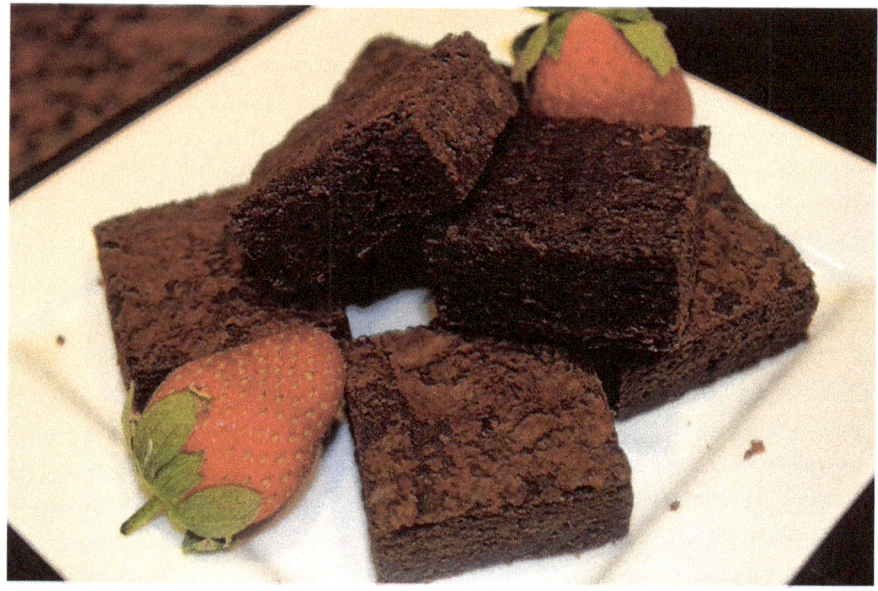

A tasty brownie, with very healthy ingredients.

Servings: 8 pieces
Preparation Time: 5 minutes
Cooking Time: 30 minutes

Ingredients:

- 1 x 14oz/400g can black beans (drained)
- 2 eggs
- 1tsp vanilla extract
- Pinch of salt
- 2oz/55g brown sugar

Method:

1. Put all the ingredients in a blender together and blend well.
2. Pour this mixture in a greased cake pan (8x8 inches/20x20cm)

3. You can mix some carob chips in at this time, if you need to, or can skip this step.
4. Place the cake pan in the oven for almost 30 minutes at 350°F/180°C/Gas mark 4.
5. Cool at room temperature before serving.
6. Cut into slices and serve.

Nutritional Values	per Brownie
Calories	112
Protein	6g
Fat	1g
Carbs	19g

DAY 4

Honey Apple Yogurt

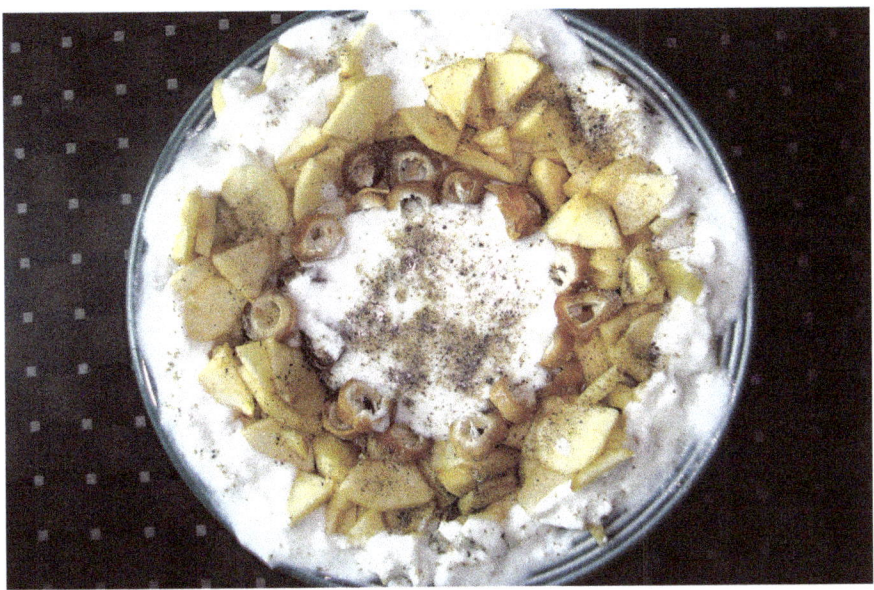

Quick and simple to make, this is a pretty delicious start to your morning. Unusually, the addition of black pepper really brings out a much deeper flavor.

Servings: 2
Preparation Time: 10 minutes
Cooking Time: No cooking required

Ingredients:

- 2tbsp raw honey
- 8fl.oz/250ml Greek Yogurt (whole milk)
- 2½oz/75g fresh crisp apples (cut into thin slices)
- 2½oz/75g dates (cut into round slices)
- ½tsp black pepper or cinnamon

Method:

1. In a bowl, mix all the ingredients together very well, except black pepper.
2. Serve on a large decorative plate and sprinkle black pepper over it.

3. You can also garnish with a few additional apple and date slices.

Enjoy!

Nutritional Values	per Serving
Calories	262
Protein	14g
Fat	<1g
Carbs	55g

Cranberry and Raspberry Smoothie

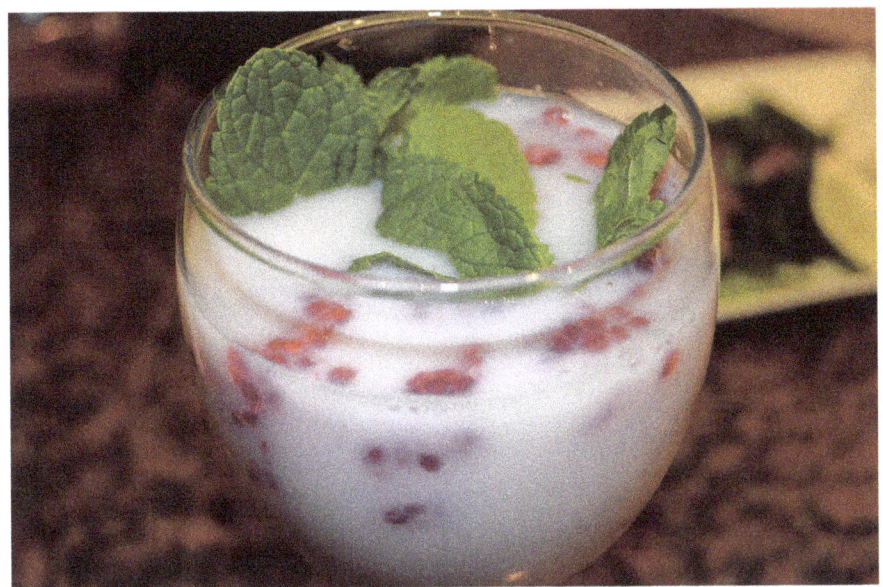

A low fat, vitamin C-packed smoothie to start your day

Servings: 4-6
Preparation Time: 10 minutes
Cooking Time: No cooking required

Ingredients:

- 200ml cranberry juice
- 175g frozen raspberries, defrosted
- 100ml milk
- 200ml natural yogurt
- 1 tbsp caster sugar, or to taste
- mint sprigs, to serve

Method:

1. Place all the ingredients into a blender and pulse until smooth.
2. Pour into glasses and serve topped with fresh mint.

Nutritional Values	per Serving
Calories	97
Protein	7g
Fat	1g
Carbs	16g

Middle Eastern Salad with Grilled Halloumi

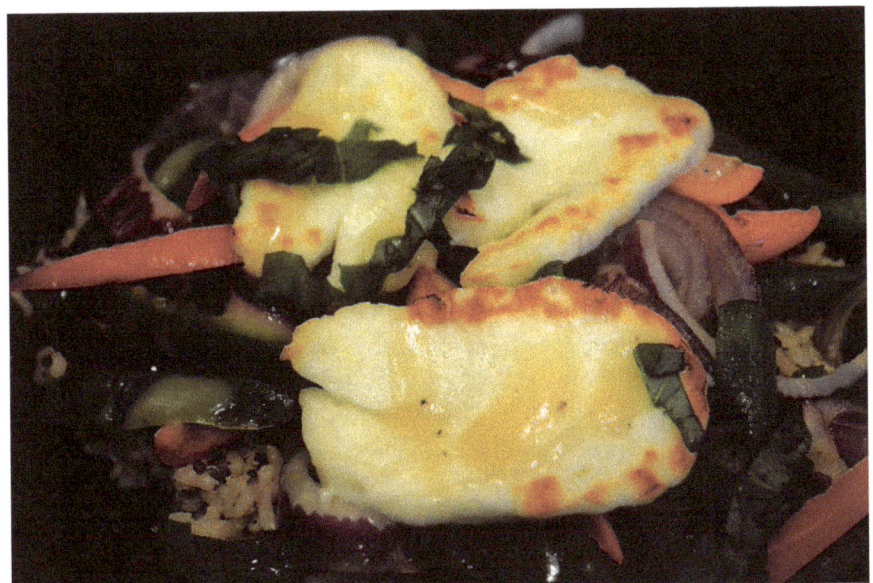

A delightful and filling dish with so many variations, but very traditional in the Middle East, Greece and Turkey.

Servings: 4
Preparation Time: 15 minutes
Cooking Time: 25 minutes

Ingredients:

- 3tbsp extra-virgin olive oil
- 1 small red onion, sliced
- 2 bell peppers (red and green for color, seeds removed and sliced
- 7oz/200g quinoa
- 16fl.oz/500ml vegetable stock
- Small bunch flat-leaf parsley, roughly chopped
- Zest and juice 1 lemon
- Zest and juice of 1 lime
- 10oz/300g halloumi cheese, cut into 8 slices
- Seasoning to taste

Method:

1. Heat 1tbsp of the oil in a medium-sized saucepan.
2. Cook the onion and pepper until just beginning to soften, then add the quinoa and cook for a further 3 minutes.
3. Add the stock, cover and turn the heat down to a simmer.
4. Cook for 10 minutes or until soft then stir through half the parsley.
5. Place the halloumi on a tray lined with foil.
6. Heat the grill to high, but put the tray on the second shelf down, not too close to the grill.
7. Meanwhile, mix the lemon zest and juice with the remaining parsley and oil, and a large pinch of pepper and salt.
8. Grill the halloumi until both sides are golden and crisp.
9. Serve the salad with the grilled halloumi on the top and the dressing poured over everything.
10. Make sure you serve up the dish immediately, as halloumi when cooling down becomes quite 'tough'.

Nutritional Values	per Serving
Calories	447
Protein	14g
Fat	25g
Carbs	44g

Salmon Scallion and Ginger Fishcakes

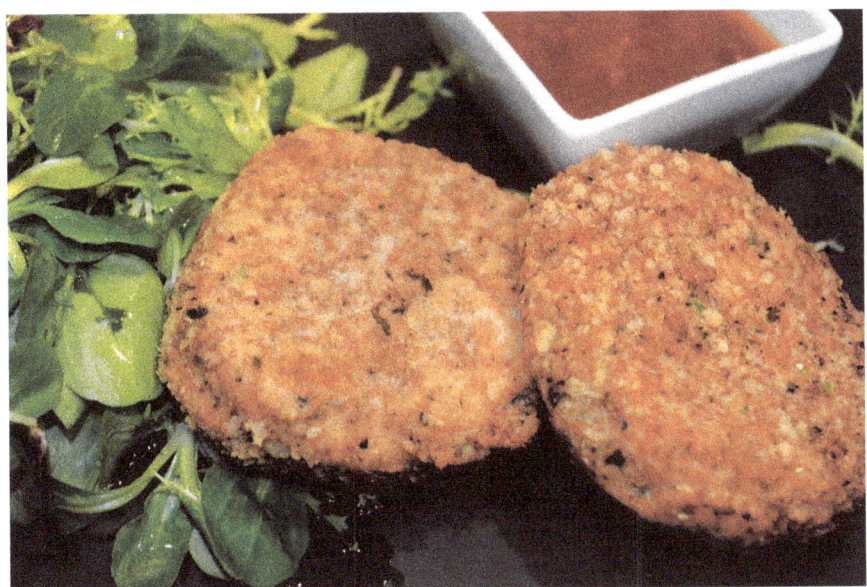

A taste of the Orient - a lovely healthy supper with these light, Asian-style fish cakes. Double the quantities if you want more!

Servings: 4 (makes 4 patties)
Preparation Time: 15 minutes
Cooking Time: 30 minutes

Ingredients:

- 2 x 5oz/140g skinless salmon fillets
- 1in/2½cm piece ginger, grated
- 1 large sweet potato, baked and flesh removed
- Zest 1 lime
- ½ bunch scallions, finely chopped
- Gluten-free flour for dusting
- 2tbsp mayonnaise mixed with wasabi (optional)
- Extra lime wedges to serve

Method:

1. Microwave the sweet potato until completely cooked through and soft in the middle. Remove flesh and place in a bowl.
2. Heat oven to 400°F/200°C/gas mark 6.
3. Chop the salmon as finely as you can and place in a bowl with the sweet potato, ginger, lime zest and seasoning.
4. Heat 1tsp oil in a non-stick pan and soften the scallions for 2 minutes. Stir into the salmon, mix well and shape into 4 patties. Dust with flour.
5. Heat remaining oil in the pan and cook the patties for 3-4 minutes each side until golden and cooked through.
6. Cover with a lid and leave to rest for a few minutes.
7. Serve 2 patties each with a mixed salad or homemade sweet potato chips, mayo and lime wedges for squeezing a zesty tang over the fishcakes.

Nutritional Values	per Serving
Calories	196
Protein	15g
Fat	10g
Carbs	12g

Lemon Tart with Fresh Blueberries

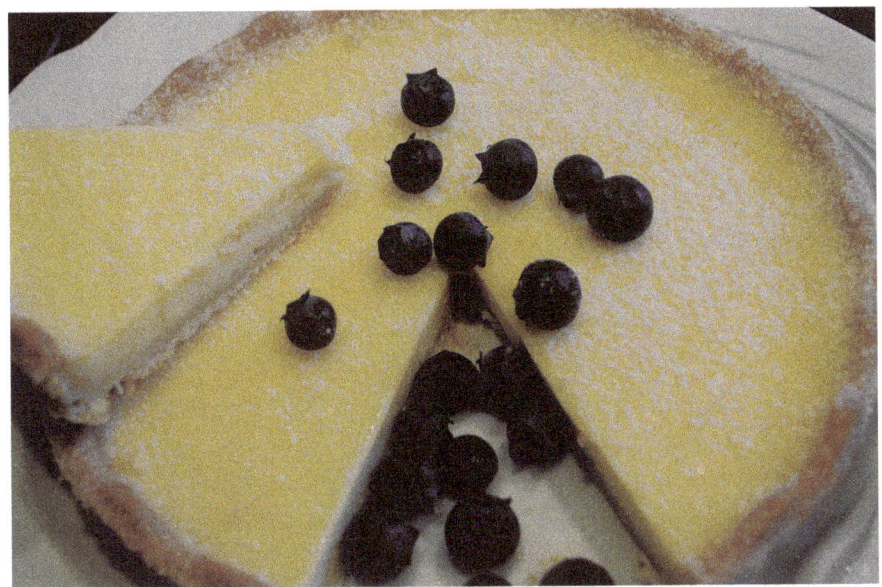

Blueberries and lemon are a classic combination, slightly sharp, but nothing a small scoop of ice cream won't cure. Make this a day in advance if you can, as it takes a little longer than most of our other recipes.

Servings: 8 portions (save some to eat as a snack)
Preparation Time: 20 minutes
Cooking Time: Approximately 1 hour

Ingredients:

For the pastry
- 10oz/300g gluten-free plain flour, and a little extra for dusting surface
- 1tsp xanthan gum
- Zest of 1 lemon
- 5oz/140g butter, cut into small cubes
- 1 egg, beaten
- 2oz/55g icing sugar (make sure it is gluten-free – some may contain gluten)

For the filling
- 5 large organic eggs
- 4½oz/125g caster sugar
- 4fl.oz/120ml thick cream
- 4fl.oz/120ml fresh lemon juice
- Zest from the lemons used for juice (should be about 2tbsp)

For the pie crust
- Parchment paper or aluminum foil
- Pie weights, dry beans, or pennies

Method:

1. Heat oven to 350°F/180°C/Gas Mark 6.
2. Using a food processor, place the flour, xanthan, lemon zest, butter and icing sugar and a pinch of salt into the bowl and whizz to a very fine crumb.
3. Beat the egg with a tablespoon of water and gradually drizzle into the processor whilst the machine is still going. It should begin to start forming a dough, but be ready to add a little more water at a time if need be.
4. Once you have a firm but kneadable dough, removed from the processor and knead for 2 minutes. Wrap in cling film and refrigerate for 30 minutes.
5. Beat the filling ingredients together (excluding the zest). Pass through a sieve and then add the zest.
6. Roll the pastry out on a lightly floured surface
7. Line your tart tin with the rolled-out pastry.
8. Once the tin is lined with your pastry, cover with the parchment paper or aluminum foil.
9. Fill with pie weights, dry beans or pennies and bake for 15 minutes.
10. Remove from the oven and gently remove the weights and paper/foil.
11. Replace in the oven and bake for a further 15 minutes until the pastry is firm to the touch.
12. Pour in the lemon mix and bake the tart for 30 minutes. This should be enough to just set the tart.
13. Leave to cool before removing from the tin.
14. This should make 8 reasonable sized portions.

Nutritional Values	per Serving
Calories	461
Protein	9g
Fat	24g
Carbs	54g

DAY 5

Easy Scrambled Eggs

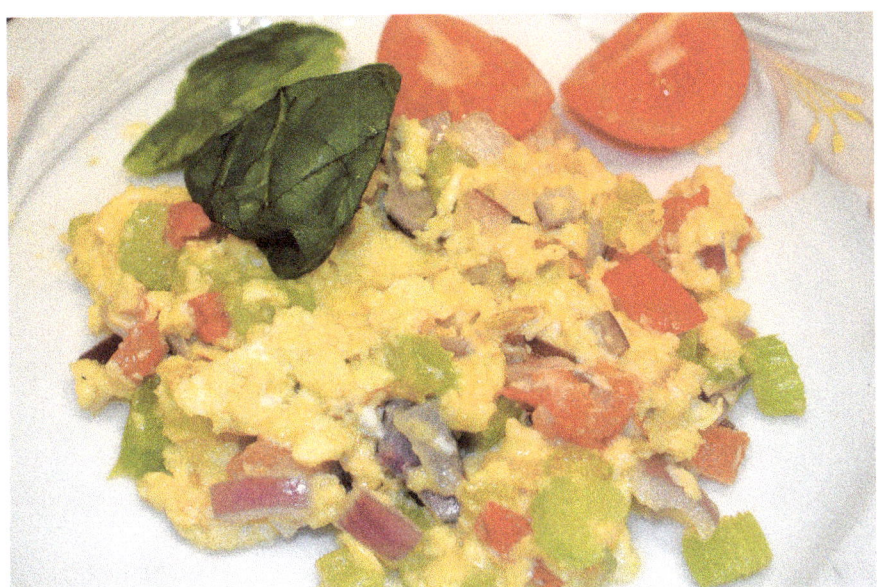

Add a twist to your scrambled eggs by giving them a little crunch. Finely diced celery makes a healthy difference to just ordinary scrambled eggs and a little spice with the pepper.

Servings: 4
Preparation Time: 10 minutes
Cooking Time: 6-8 minutes

Ingredients:

- 2tbsp butter
- 8 eggs
- 1 red onion
- 2 celery sticks, finely diced
- 1 large tomato (chopped)
- pinch of cumin seeds
- ½tsp salt
- ½tsp black pepper
- 2tbsp water
- herbs to garnish

Method:

1. In a bowl, beat eggs with salt and water.
2. In a skillet, melt butter on medium heat.
3. Add chopped onion and celery and cook for 3-5 minutes. Then add tomatoes mixing continuously till tender.
4. When the vegetable mix is tender, add egg mixture, cumin seeds and black pepper.
5. Let them cook mixing constantly till eggs are to your liking.
6. Garnish with coriander leaves or fresh parsley and serve.

Nutritional Values	per Serving
Calories	224
Protein	14g
Fat	16g
Carbs	7g

Sausage Rolls with a Kick!

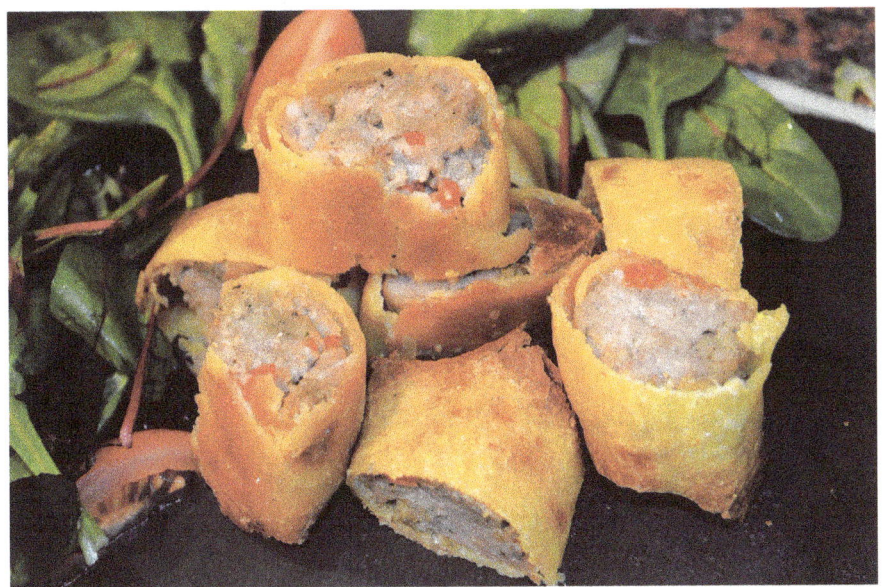

If you like your sausage rolls with a little bit of a herby kick then these gluten-free treats are for you.

Servings: Makes 16 sausage rolls
Preparation Time: 10 minutes
Cooking Time: 20 minutes

Ingredients:

- 1 block gluten-free puff pastry (8oz/225g)
- 8 gluten-free sausages
- 1tbsp finely parsley, finely chopped
- 1tsp sage, finely chopped
- 1 red chillies, very finely chopped
- Seasoning (plenty of pepper!)
- 1 egg, beaten

Method:

1. Roll the puff pastry out to a rectangle approximately 20x12inch or 45x30cm.
2. Take the sausage meat out of the skins of the sausages.

3. Mix in the herbs, chillies and seasoning. Make sure it is thoroughly combined.
4. Spread sausage meat over pastry, leaving a little rim round the edge.
5. Brush with beaten egg.
6. Fold the pastry over, seal and glaze.
7. Cut into even pieces, whatever size you want (16 is a good number).
8. Place onto a non-stick baking sheet, brush with the egg and bake for 15 minutes at 400°F/200°C/Gas mark 6.
9. Leave to cool a little and serve.

Nutritional Values	per Serving (1 roll)
Calories	96
Protein	5g
Fat	7g
Carbs	4g

Pancetta and Polenta Bake

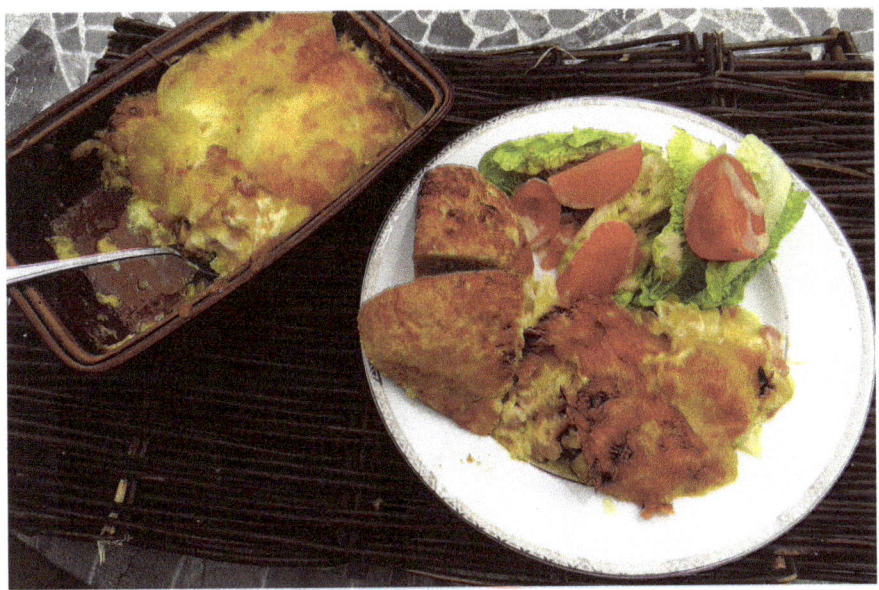

Based on a traditional French recipe but using polenta instead of potatoes, just for a different texture and taste! You could use this as a side dish with meat, but it is delightful as a main course at lunch or brunch with a tossed salad.

Servings: 4 portions
Preparation Time: 10 minutes
Cooking Time: 40 minutes

Ingredients:

- 2tbsp olive oil
- 5oz/140g pancetta or lardons (cubed)
- 1 small onion, diced
- 2 cloves garlic, crushed
- 2tbsp fresh thyme leaves
- 2oz/55g fresh Parmesan cheese, grated
- 5fl.oz/150ml single cream
- 5fl.oz/150ml fresh gluten-free chicken stock, or made with gluten-free stock cubes and water
- 9oz/250g ready cooked polenta, cut into cubes

Method:

1. Heat oven to 400°F/200°C/Gas mark 6.
2. Prepare a baking dish by lightly oiling.
3. Using a large skillet or frying pan, sauté the onion in the olive oil until soft but not mushy.
4. Mix in the pancetta or lardons, garlic and thyme leaves. Make sure the pancetta or lardons get slightly crispy.
5. Mix in the polenta and some of the Parmesan (you need to leave some for sprinkling over the top) and cook for 2-3 minutes.
6. Add stock and cream to the skillet, stir to mix thoroughly before pouring the whole mix into the baking dish.
7. Sprinkle with the remaining Parmesan and bake for approximately 40 minutes until lightly golden brown on the top.
8. Serve with a delicious mixed salad.

Nutritional Values	per Serving
Calories	366
Protein	11g
Fat	29g
Carbs	16g

Oriental Lamb Stir Fry

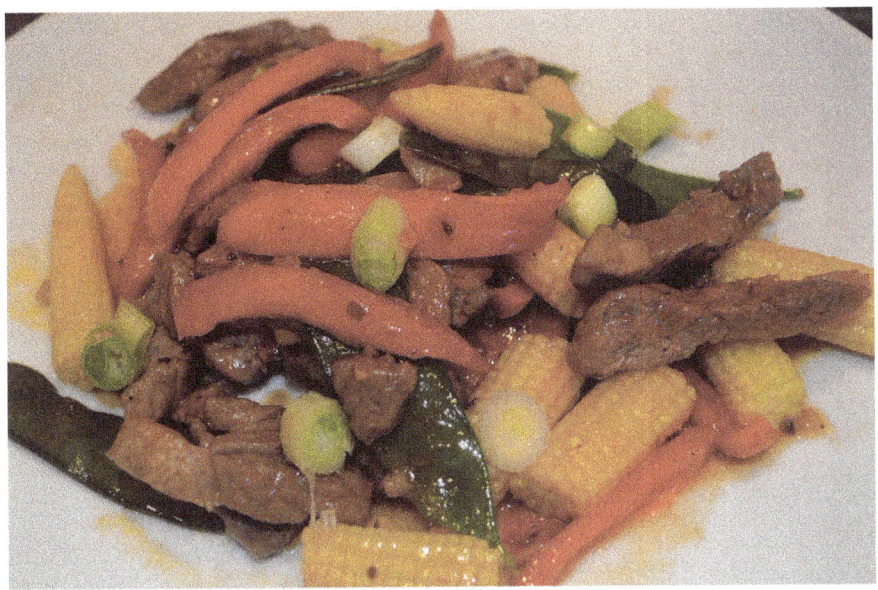

A very quick and easy dish, prepare the marinade and soak the sliced lamb steak at least 2 hours before cooking. Chop the vegetables at the same time and refrigerate in an airtight box – then cook the meal in a couple of minutes!

Servings: 4
Preparation time: 10 minutes (plus time to marinade)
Cooking time: 5 minutes

Ingredients:

- 1lb/450g lamb steak, sliced
- 1 red pepper, sliced
- 1 bunch spring onions (scallions), chopped (including greens)
- 8oz/225g baby sweetcorn
- 8oz/225g mange tout peas
- 8oz/225g bean sprouts
- 2tbsp sesame oil, to fry

For the marinade

- 4tbsp peanut butter
- 4tbsp light wheat-free soy or tamari sauce

- 4tbsp sherry (or a sweet dessert wine)
- Juice and zest of a lime
- 2 garlic cloves, minced
- 1inch/2cm ginger, peeled and finely chopped
- 8tbsp water

Method:

1. Mix all marinade ingredients in a large bowl.
2. Add lamb pieces and cover. Refrigerate for at least 2 hours.
3. Heat sesame oil in a wok or large frying pan.
4. Remove lamb from marinade and fry for 2-3 minutes. Remove from pan.
5. Add peppers and spring onion to pan, fry for 1 minute.
6. Add mange tout and sweetcorn, fry for another minute.
7. Pour marinade in and allow to reduce down slightly.
8. Stir in beansprouts and lamb, heat through and serve.

Nutritional Values	per Serving
Calories	627
Protein	29g
Fat	46g
Carbs	23g

Mango and Papaya Fool

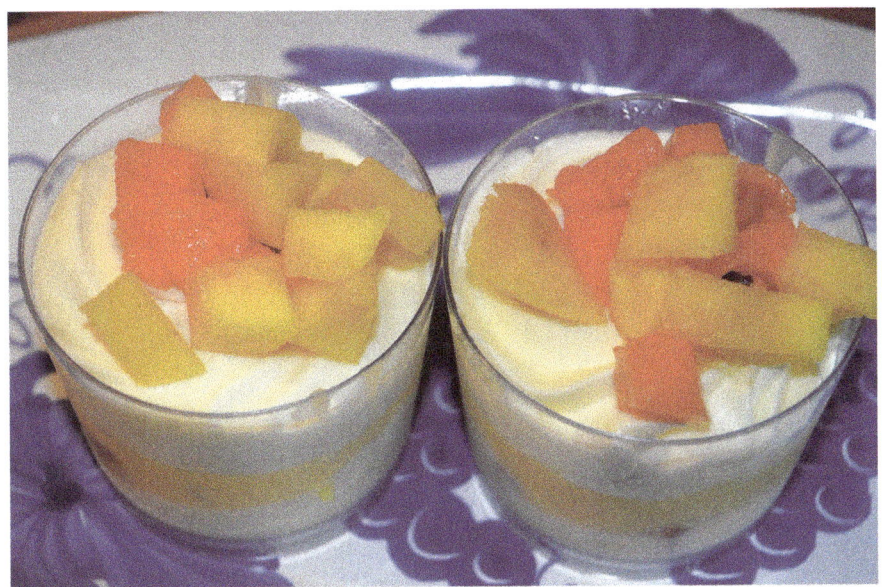

This is a delicious sweet but sharp dessert, low in calories and fat. You could also eat this for breakfast, if desired.

Servings: 4
Preparation Time: 10 minutes
Cooking Time: No cooking required

Ingredients:

- 1 large mango, peeled, de-stoned and diced
- 1 large papaya, peeled and diced
- 150mls low fat Greek Yogurt
- Juice of 1 lime

Method:

1. Simply divide the yogurt among 4 small glasses or pots.
2. Top with the diced mango and papaya.
3. Squeeze over the lime juice.
4. If required, drizzle a little honey over the top (will add to calories, but not much).
5. Serve cold from the fridge.

Nutritional Values	per Serving
Calories	154
Protein	4g
Fat	1g
Carbs	36g

DAY 6

Stuffed Herb Mushrooms

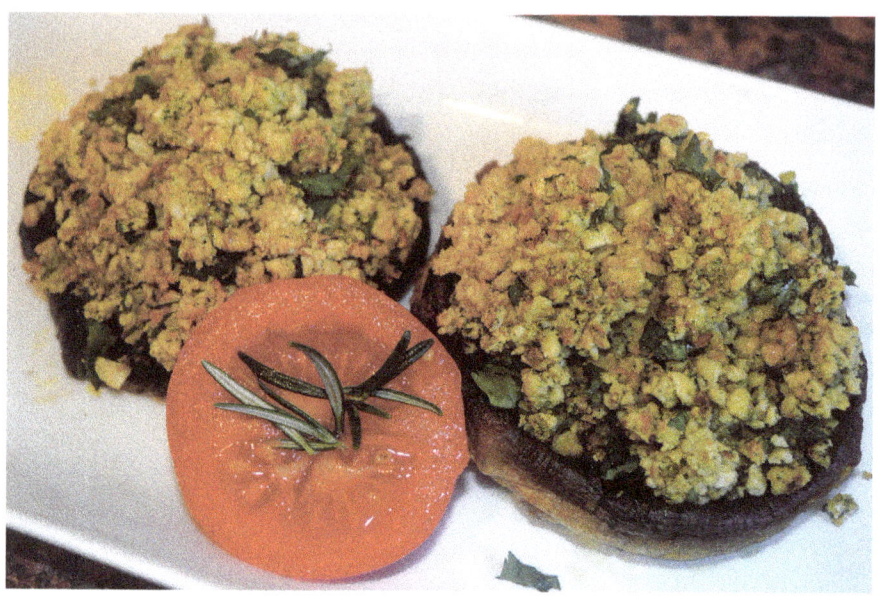

This dish is delicious as a breakfast served with tasty gluten-free bread to mop up the juices, or as light meal with salad.

Servings: 4
Preparation Time: Less than 30 minutes
Cooking Time: 15 minutes

Ingredients:

- 4oz/115g (dairy free) butter, softened
- 8 large flat mushrooms, stems removed and finely chopped
- 3½oz/100g fresh white gluten-free breadcrumbs
- 1tbsp chopped thyme
- 1tbsp chopped parsley
- Zest of 1 lemon
- Salt and pepper
- 1 egg, lightly beaten

- 2 cloves garlic, crushed (optional)

Method:

1. Preheat the oven to 350°F/180°C/Gas mark 4.
2. Arrange the mushroom caps, top down on a baking sheet.
3. Beat the garlic into the butter and divide 2/3 of the butter among the mushroom caps.
4. Melt the remaining butter in a pan and add the breadcrumbs. Gently fry until golden then tip into a bowl.
5. Stir in the thyme, parsley, lemon zest, chopped mushroom stems and season to taste with salt and pepper. Stir in the beaten egg.
6. Divide the breadcrumb mixture evenly among the mushroom caps.
7. Bake for 15 minutes or until the stuffing is golden brown and the mushrooms are tender.
8. Serve immediately with or without the bread to mop up the juices.

Nutritional Values	per Serving
Calories	319
Protein	6g
Fat	25g
Carbs	20g

Fig and Pistachio Flapjacks

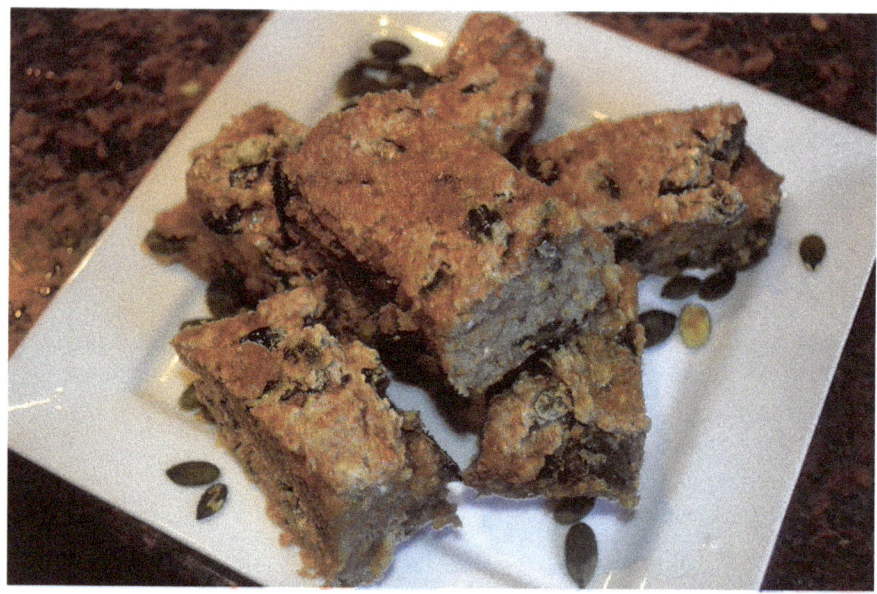

Great little snack bars you can have as a morning coffee treat, afternoon tea or take in the car with you for that 'munchy moment'.

Servings: 16 small bars
Preparation Time: 5-10 minutes
Cooking Time: 30 minutes (plus 5 minutes with oven off)

Ingredients:

- 5oz/140g dried figs (you could also use dried apricots or other dried fruit)
- 6oz/170g gluten-free rolled oats
- 3oz/85g pistachio nuts, roughly chopped
- 3tbsp honey or maple syrup
- 6oz/170g soft brown sugar
- 6oz/170g butter

Method:

1. Heat oven to 325°F/160°C/Gas mark 3.
2. Prepare a square baking dish (approximately 8in/20cm) by greasing and lining with parchment paper.
3. Place the butter, sugar and honey or syrup in a pan and heat gently until the mix has melted all together.
4. Put the oats, chopped nuts and figs into a bowl and pour over the melted butter mix. Stir thoroughly to combine.
5. Pour the mix into the lined baking dish and pop into the oven.
6. Bake for 30-35 minutes, then turn off the oven and leave the dish inside for 5 minutes.
7. Remove from the oven and leave to cool before slicing into required size bars.
8. Store in a clip top box or tin – they will stay fine for up to 5 days.

Nutritional Values	per Bar
Calories	199
Protein	2.3g
Fat	11.3g
Carbs	24g

Lemon and Herb Salmon

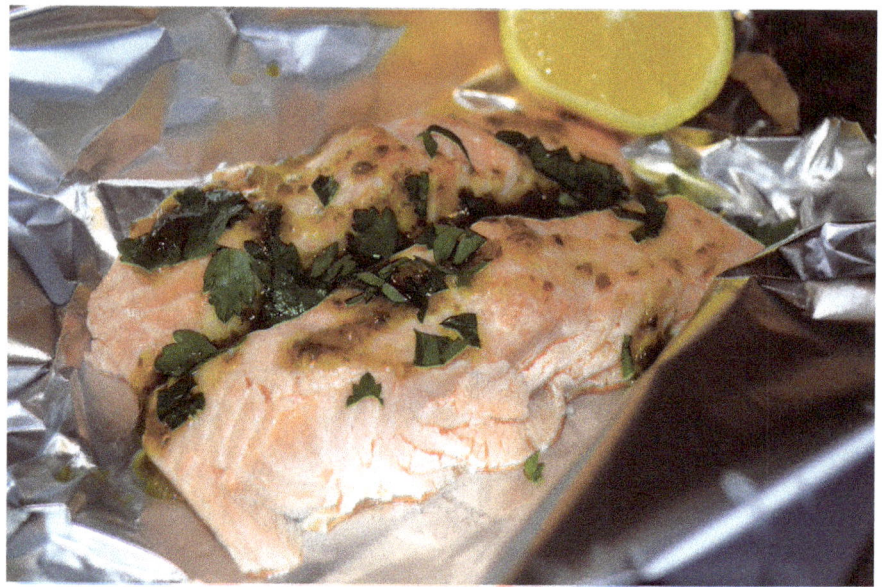

Super Salmon – one of the healthiest foods you can eat, full of Omega-3 healthy fat that comes from oily fish. Salmon should be served in a fairly simple fashion and then complemented by the vegetables or a salad.

Servings: 4
Preparation Time: 10 minutes
CookTime: 10 minutes

Ingredients:

- Olive oil as required
- 4 x salmon fillets (approximately 4oz/115g each)
- 2tbsp lemon juice
- Salt and red pepper flakes to taste
- 1tbsp fresh dill, finely chopped

Method:

1. Marinate salmon fillets with lemon, salt, and pepper for 15 minutes.
2. In a pan, heat the oil and put the salmon into it with skin side down.
3. Cook till brown and then turn over the side.
4. Cook on very low heat until the salmon is cooked all the way through (about 5-7 minutes).
5. Sprinkle over lemon juice, dill and some more seasoning. You could use parsley as an alternative.
6. Try serving with stir-fried broccoli and bell peppers to add a crunchy texture.

Nutritional Values	per Serving
Calories	226
Protein	23g
Fat	14g
Carbs	1g

One Pot Beef Stew

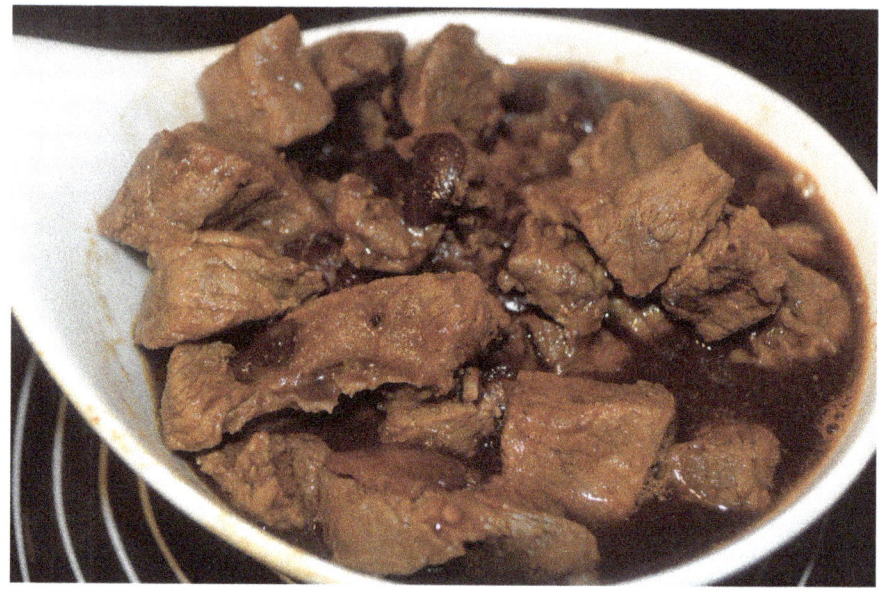

A rich and chunky stew. Prepare it, put it in the oven, and get on with something else for a couple of hours while your kitchen fills with gorgeous aromas.

Servings: 4
Preparation time: 10 minutes
Cooking time: 2 hours

Ingredients:

- 1lb/450g stewing beef, cut into chunks
- 2 carrots, sliced
- 2 onions, sliced
- 2 celery stalks, sliced
- 2 large potatoes, cut into 1inch/2cm chunks
- 3oz/85g GF flour, to coat meat
- 1 pint beef stock
- 8fl.oz/240ml red wine

- 1tsp dried oregano
- 1tsp dried thyme
- 2 bay leaves
- Salt and pepper

Method:

1. Preheat oven to 350°F/180°C/ gas mark 4.
2. Put flour, salt and pepper into a plastic zip lock bag.
3. Add chunks of beef, seal bag and shake well to coat meat.
4. Chop vegetables into chunks.
5. Place all ingredients into an oven proof dish, mixing well.
6. Cook in oven for 2 hours, or until meat is tender and gravy has thickened.
7. Season to taste.
8. Remove bay leaves before serving.

Nutritional Values	per Serving
Calories	377
Protein	9g
Fat	2g
Carbs	68g

Mixed Berry Bake

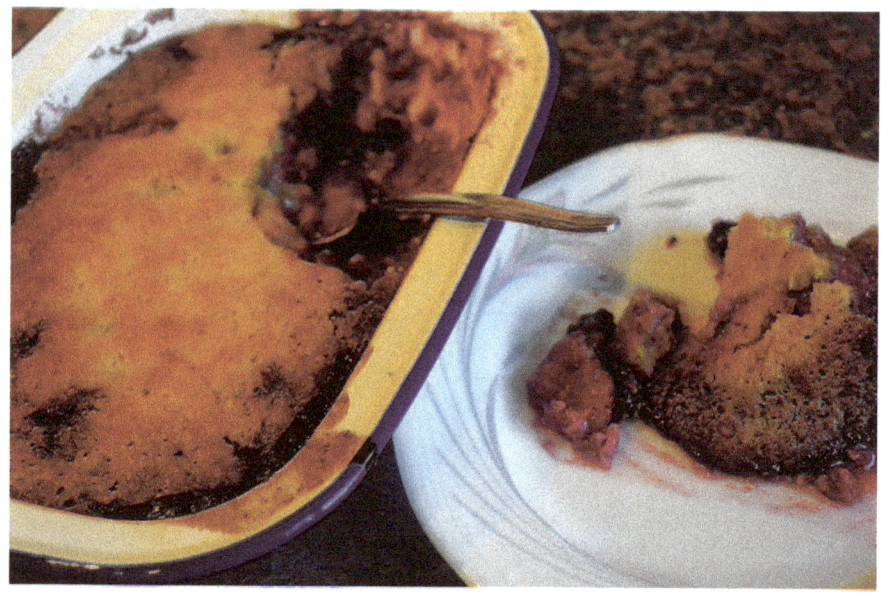

Another easy recipe, particularly if you use frozen berries, which are always a great asset in your freezer for all types of dishes.

Servings: 4
Preparation Time: 10 minutes
Cooking Time: 35-40 minutes

Ingredients:

- 1¾lb/800g mixed berries (frozen)
- 4oz/115g butter
- A little more butter for greasing
- 4oz/115g caster sugar
- 4oz/115g gluten-free flour
- 1tsp gluten-free baking powder
- 2 large eggs
- 1tsp vanilla extract
- 1tsp cinnamon

- 1oz/25g flaked almonds or other nuts that you enjoy

Method:

1. Heat oven to 350°F/180°C/Gas Mark 4.
2. Grease a square baking dish (approx. 10inx10in/25cmx25cm) and pour in the frozen berries. Add a little sugar if required.
3. Using a food processor, blend together the flour, butter, sugar, baking powder and eggs.
4. Add the vanilla extract and mix until thoroughly smooth.
5. Pour or spoon the cake mix over the berries and scatter over the almonds or nuts.
6. Bake for 35-40 minutes until risen and cooked through. Some of the berry mix may come up to the top, but that just adds to the delight of this dessert!
7. Try serving with ice cream or if you prefer, mascarpone cheese.

Nutritional Values	per Serving
Calories	616
Protein	9g
Fat	33g
Carbs	76g

DAY 7

Cheesy Scones

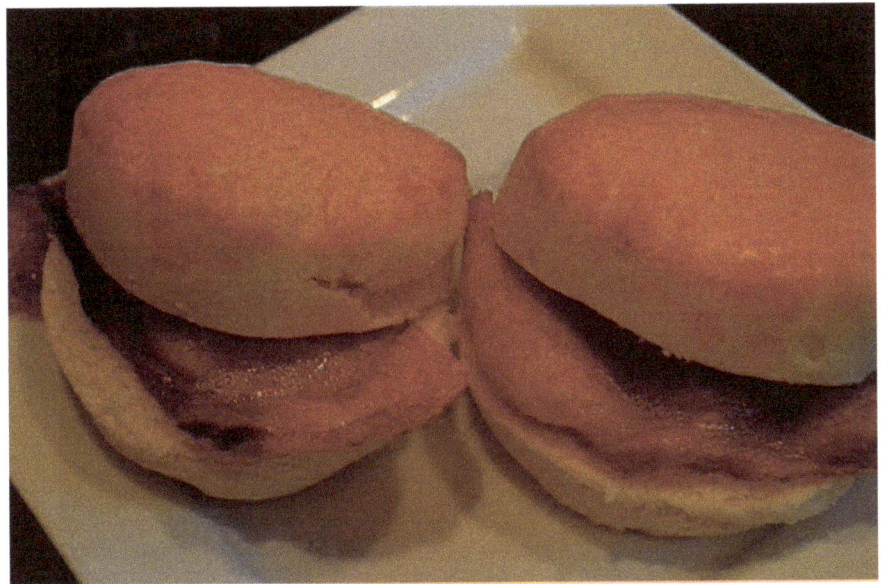

Warm cheese scones are delicious at breakfast time, or great for a snack. You could also use them as part of breakfast with some grilled bacon.

Servings: 8 scones
Preparation Time: 20 minutes
Cooking Time: 15 minutes

Ingredients:

- 7oz/200g gluten-free all-purpose flour
- Extra flour for dusting
- 1tsp bicarbonate of soda
- 8tbsp milk or buttermilk
- 1 egg, beaten
- 2oz/55g butter, cubed (take butter straight from the fridge so that it is cold)
- 4oz/115g cheddar or 2oz/55g cheddar and 2oz/55g Parmesan (extra cheesy taste if you combine)

Method:

1. Heat oven to 400°F/200°C/Gas mark 6.
2. Line a baking sheet with parchment paper.
3. Using a food processor and a sifter, sift the flour and bicarbonate of soda into the bowl. Add butter and blitz until the mixture resembles breadcrumbs.
4. Take the bowl away from the processor and mix in the cheese and the milk. This should form a slightly sticky but firm dough.
5. Lightly flour your work surface, bring the dough around and then flatten with your hands (you can use a rolling pin, but you must not overwork the dough). The dough should be around 1¼inches/3cm thick.
6. Cut rounds out of the dough with a simple or fluted cutter, approximately 3in/7cm in size. Any spare bits of dough can be scraped up and molded again for extra scones.
7. Put the scones onto the baking tray and brush with egg wash.
8. If required you can use a little extra cheese on the tops for more flavor.
9. Bake for 15 minutes until tops are golden brown and the scones are firm.
10. Scones can be frozen if you want.

Nutritional Values	per Scone
Calories	230
Protein	8g
Fat	13g
Carbs	22g

Provence Pizza

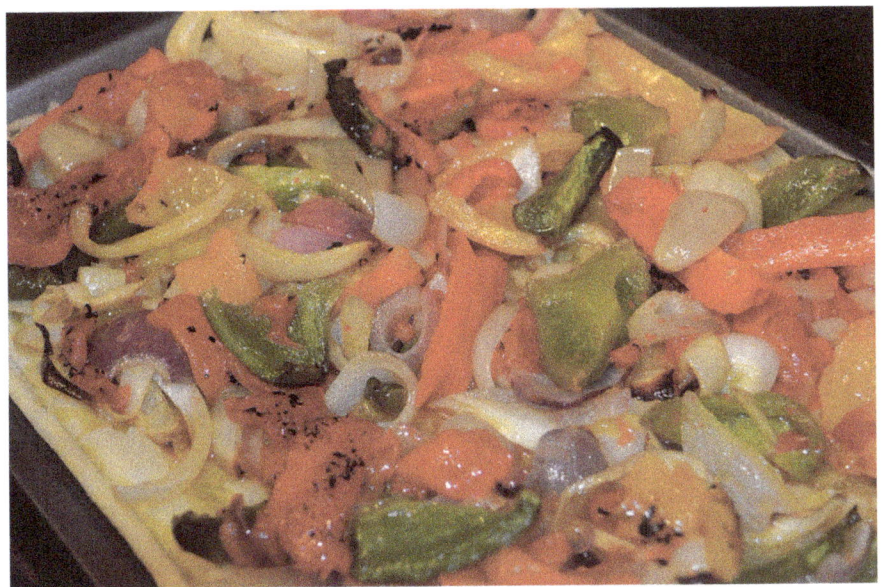

We love this recipe – apart from making the pizza dough, it is fun to make, tastes lovely and will certainly be a hit with all the family. You could vary the toppings with vegetables to suit, but this one gives a real hint of the South of France.

Servings: 4
Preparation Time: 45 minutes (plus rising time for dough)
Cooking Time: 1 hour

Ingredients:

For the dough
- 1lb/450g gluten-free plain flour, plus extra for dusting surface
- 1 x ¼oz/7g sachet fast action yeast
- 2 eggs beaten
- 1tsp fine (caster) sugar
- 1tsp xanthan gum
- Olive oil (about 6tbsp)

For the topping
- 4tbsp olive oil
- 2 large sweet white onions, or 3 medium size red onions
- 4 bell peppers, mixed colors (makes the pizza look lovely!), seeds removed and sliced
- 3 cloves garlic, finely sliced or very finely chopped
- 1tbsp cornichons (baby gherkins) finely sliced
- 5 or 6tbsp pitted black olives (or you can use green) sliced

Method:

1. Heat oven to 350°F/180°C/Gas Mark 6.
2. Take a large baking tray and place all the raw vegetables (onions, garlic, peppers) into the tray. Pour over the olive oil, mix through and place in the oven to roast for around 40 minutes. Turn over the vegetables 3 or 4 times to prevent burning.
3. Whilst the vegetables are cooking, make the pizza dough. Use a large bowl (make sure you have a wooden spoon in hand as well) and mix the flour, sugar, xanthan, yeast and a large pinch of salt in the bowl. Mix around then make a well in the centre of the flour mix.
4. Add the beaten eggs, oil and a little water and use the wooden spoon to stir the mixture until it forms a sticky dough.
5. Flour your work surface, remove the dough from the bowl and knead for around 5 minutes with firm movements. Place in an oiled bowl, cover with a clean tea cloth and keep in a warm place for a further 25-30 minutes until the dough has risen.
6. While the dough is rising, prepare a 16x12inch/40x30cm baking sheet by lightly greasing it with a little olive oil (very lightly). Roll out the dough so that it fits just inside the baking sheet.
7. Spoon over your roasted topping mix, scatter with the cornichons and olives. Place into the oven and bake for 20-25 minutes until the dough has risen nicely and cooked through.
8. Scatter over some fresh chopped basil and a little more olive oil if required – you are now in Provence!

Nutritional Values	per Serving
Calories	655
Protein	16g
Fat	28g
Carbs	87g

Homemade Savory Crackers

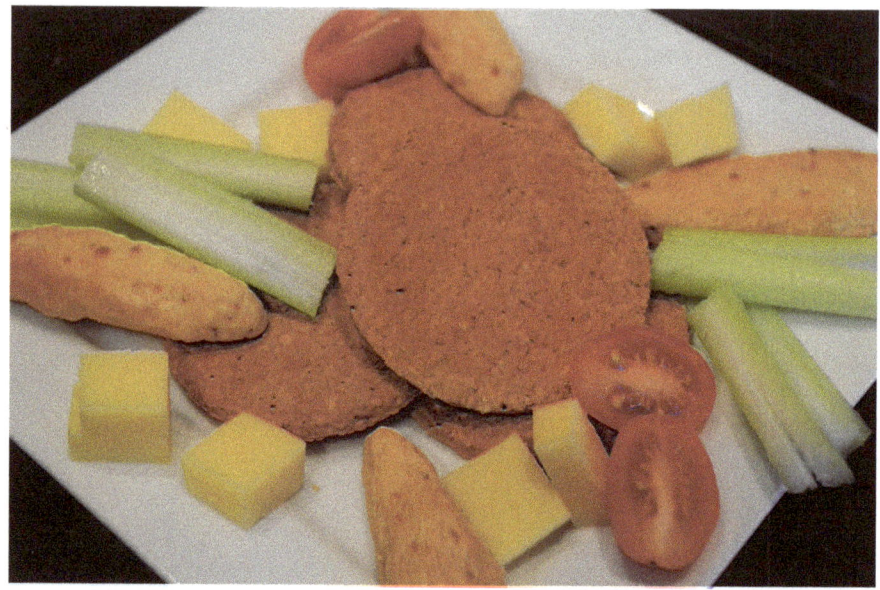

These crackers are so tasty that you could eat them on their own! Really useful to have around and stop temptation to reach for anything from the cupboard. Delicious with more cheese, coleslaw, dips and more. The recipe below makes quite a lot of crackers depending on the size you cut them, so you could halve the recipe and keep the remaining dough in the fridge for use a few days later, to top up your supply!

Servings: 50 medium size crackers
Preparation Time: 20 minutes
Cooking Time: 20 minutes

Ingredients:

- 7oz/200g gluten-free all-purpose flour
- 1tsp salt
- A few grinds of black pepper
- 1tsp ground chia seeds

- ½tsp dried rosemary or Provence herbs (your preference)
- 3tbsp cold unsalted butter, cut into small cubes
- 6oz/170g strong cheddar cheese, grated (or half cheddar, half Parmesan)
- 1tsp Dijon mustard (check label for gluten-free)
- 2tsp apple cider vinegar
- Ice cold water, to hand

Method:

1. Heat oven to 350°F/180°C/Gas Mark 4.
2. Mix all the dry ingredients together, either using your hands or in the food processor.
3. Drop the butter cubes into the mix and pulse in the processor until the butter has divided into very small chunks in the mixture. This is probably pulsing around 6 times.
4. Add the cheese and the mustard and pulse again.
5. Add the apple cider vinegar and 4tbsp of iced water and pulse again. Have a look and see how far you are away from a nice ball of dough.
6. Continue to add water until the dough forms a ball.
7. Wrap in plastic wrap and place in the fridge, preferably overnight, but for at least 2 hours.
8. Line a baking sheet with parchment paper to prepare for placing the cut out crackers onto it.
9. Tear off two more pieces of parchment paper and place the dough in between them. Roll out the dough to about 1/8 inch/3mm thick (as thin as you can get before it is impossible to handle!) and using a medium sized round, square or rectangular cutter, cut out the cracker shapes.
10. Slide the crackers onto the baking sheet and pop into the oven.
11. Bake the crackers for around 20 minutes until a light golden colour.
12. Remove from the oven and leave to cool (they will harden up whilst cooling).
13. When completely cool, place in an airtight container for storage.

Nutritional Values	per Cracker
Calories	37
Protein	1g
Fat	2g
Carbs	3g

Chinese Pork Tenderloin with Braised Cabbage and Leek

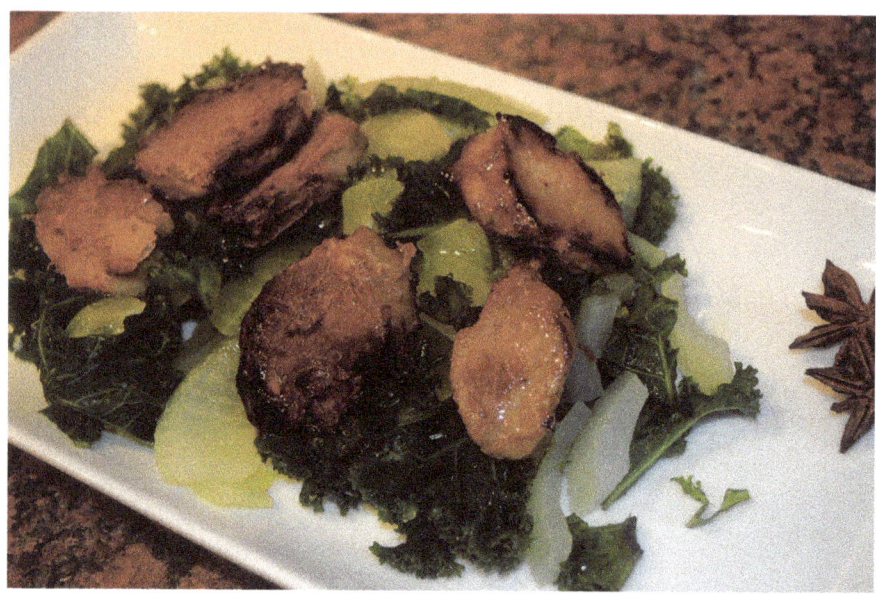

A tasty joint of pork tenderloin marinated in Chinese spices. Enjoy the flavors of the East.

Servings: 4
Preparation time: 15 minutes (plus time to marinate)
Cooking time: 1 – 1½ hours

Ingredients:

- 1½lb/675g pork tenderloin, rolled

For the marinade
- 2tbsp wheat-free soy or tamari sauce
- 4 shallots, minced/finely chopped
- 3 garlic cloves, minced
- 1tsp Chinese five-spice powder
- 1tbsp honey

For the cabbage
- 1tbsp olive oil
- ¼ cup dry white wine
- 1 large leek, sliced
- 1 green cabbage, shredded

Method:
1. Combine the marinade ingredients in a dish, mixing well.
2. Add tenderloin, rub marinade in well. Cover and refrigerate for several hours, or overnight.

To cook pork
3. Preheat oven to 400°F/200°C/gas mark 6
4. Heat oil in a frying pan.
5. Fry tenderloin in a little olive oil to seal the outside.
6. Transfer tenderloin to ovenproof dish, add 1tbsp of water, cover and place in oven for 1 – 1½ hours, or until just cooked through.

To cook cabbage
7. Heat oil in frying pan. Fry leeks to soften.
8. Add white wine, cook at high heat for a minute to burn alcohol off.
9. Turn down heat and add cabbage.
10. Cover and cook for 5 minutes.
11. Season with black pepper.

To finish off
12. When pork is cooked, remove from oven and stand for 10 minutes.
13. Slice and serve on a bed of the braised cabbage and leeks.

Nutritional Values	per Serving
Calories	369
Protein	41g
Fat	8g
Carbs	33g

No Bake Coconut Cookies

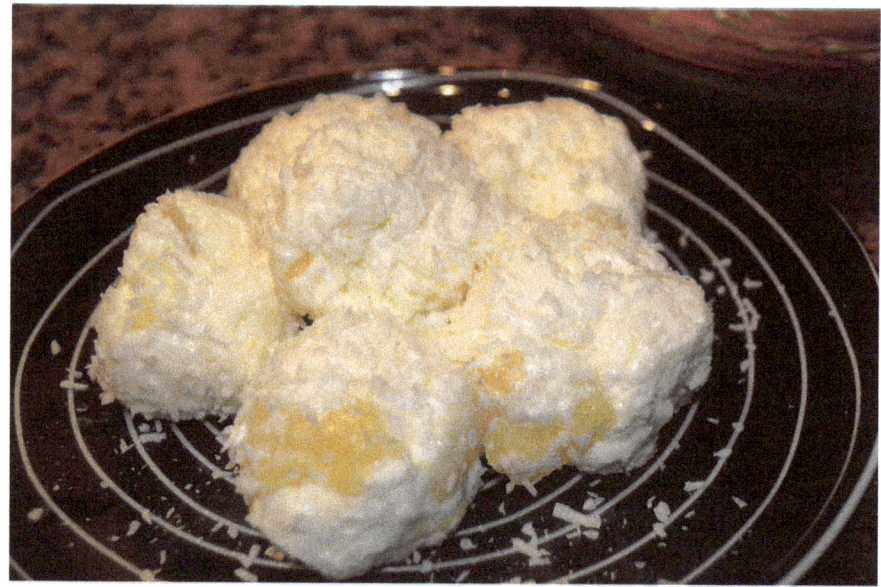

Here is an incredibly quick and easy snack to make that benefits from sitting in the fridge for a couple of hours. You can either make them in balls, or flatten them for a more cookie-like shape. Either way, we bet you will love them!

Servings: 24 cookies
Preparation Time: 10 minutes
Cooking Time: No cooking required

Ingredients:

- 12oz/340g crushed pineapple - drained (if you like them really full of pineapple, add more)
- 1lb/450g cream cheese - softened
- 1lb/450g coconut flakes

Method:

1. Drain the pineapple well using a strainer.
2. In a medium bowl, beat cream cheese and add pineapple.
3. If you are making 'cookies,' mix in all the coconut. Stir very well, cover, and put in refrigerator for 35 minutes.
4. If you are making balls, form the balls in your hands and then roll in the coconut – they look like pretty snowballs!
5. Refrigerate for 2 hours or more, then bite into these delicious morsels – yummy!

Nutritional Values	per Serving
Calories	195
Protein	2g
Fat	19g
Carbs	7g

Thank You!

If you enjoyed the meal plan, please consider leaving a review of the book. Good reviews encourage an author to write as well as help books to sell. Good reviews can be just a few short sentences describing what you liked about the book. If you could spend 30 seconds writing a review, I would appreciate it. You can review this title right now at your favorite retailer.

As a perk for purchasing this book, you can get two additional recipes (Braised Lamb Shanks with Butternut Squash and Gluten-Free Flour Mix), a printable meal plan and shopping list by signing up for my newsletter at the following the link below:

https://gotorecipecookbooks.com/gluten-free-1/

Other Books by Rachel Richards

- The 7-Day Ketogenic Diet Meal Plan: 35 Delicious Low Carb Recipes For Weight Loss Motivation - Volume 1

- The 7-Day Ketogenic Diet Meal Plan: 35 Delicious Low Carb Recipes For Weight Loss Motivation - Volume 2

- The 7-Day Ketogenic Diet Meal Plan: 35 Delicious Low Carb Recipes For Weight Loss Motivation - Volume 3

- The 7-Day Ketogenic Diet Meal Plan: 35 Delicious Low Carb Recipes For Weight Loss Motivation - Volumes 1 to 3

- 50 Vegan Slow Cooker Recipes: Delicious Meatless Slow Cooker Meals For The Vegan Lifestyle

Get the latest update on new releases from the author at:

https://rachelrichardsrecipebooks.com/newsletter/

About the Author – Rachel Richards

Rachel Richards enjoys creating specialized cookbooks for those who are health-conscious.

Visit Rachel's website at:

https://rachelrichardsrecipebooks.com/

Connect with Rachel Richards

I really appreciate you reading my book! Here are my social media contact information:

Friend me on Facebook:
https://www.facebook.com/rachelrichardsrecipebooks

Follow me on Twitter: https://twitter.com/rachlrichards

Check me out on Goodreads:
https://www.goodreads.com/author/show/14172765.Rachel_Richards

Subscribe to my newsletter:
https://rachelrichardsrecipebooks.com/newsletter/

Visit my website: https://rachelrichardsrecipebooks.com/

www.ingramcontent.com/pod-product-compliance
Lightning Source LLC
Chambersburg PA
CBHW061803070526
44586CB00023B/2696